Acupressure and Reflextherapy in the Treatment of Medical Conditions

Commissioning editor: Heidi Allen
Development editor: Robert Edwards
Production controller: Anthony Read
Desk editor: Jackie Holding
Cover designer: Gregory Harris

Acupressure and Reflextherapy in the Treatment of Medical Conditions

John R. Cross
Dr Ac., MCSP, SRP, MBAcC, MRSH

With a Foreword by James L. Oschman, PhD

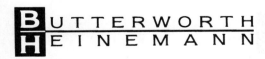

OXFORD   AUCKLAND   BOSTON   JOHANNESBURG   MELBOURNE   NEW DELHI

Butterworth-Heinemann
Linacre House, Jordan Hill, Oxford OX2 8DP
225 Wildwood Avenue, Woburn, MA 01801-2041
A division of Reed Educational and Professional Publishing Ltd

ℛ A member of the Reed Elsevier plc group

First published 2001

British Library Cataloguing in Publication Data
Cross, John R.
  Acupressure and reflextherapy in the treatment of medical conditions
  1. Acupressure   2.   Reflextherapy
  I.   Title
  615.8'22

ISBN 0 7506 4962 3

Typeset by E & M Graphics, Midsomer Norton, Bath
Printed and bound in Great Britain by Antony Rowe Ltd, Chippenham, Wiltshire

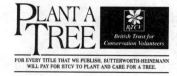

FOR EVERY TITLE THAT WE PUBLISH, BUTTERWORTH-HEINEMANN
WILL PAY FOR BTCV TO PLANT AND CARE FOR A TREE.

Contents

Foreword

We live in a time when a patient's options for successful medical treatment are expanding rapidly. This is happening because of the efforts of creative thinkers and practitioners such as John Cross. These are individuals who are never satisfied that their work is complete. They are continually advancing the theory and practice of their techniques, making them more effective, applying them to more and more clinical conditions, making them easier to practice and easier to learn. As long as anyone suffers from a seemingly intractable or incurable disorder, their job of invention and innovation is not over.

I am fascinated with the work of these pioneers who we are blessed to have among us, and upon whom the future evolution of our medicine and our species, depends. In common with a small number of other innovators, John Cross is expanding our understanding of what is involved in touch (in its many forms) and how touch relates to the overall picture of the patient – a picture that goes far beyond relieving a particular symptom. His emphasis is on information flowing in both directions, from practitioner to patient and back again, in a closed loop of sensitive and caring connections.

> What is happening all the time is that data is being traded back and forth, democratically, responsibly and cooperatively, between every cell and every membrane and every molecule. This energetic miracle of mutual nourishment is the perfect model for all of our endeavors. It is a miracle to emulate in all of our actions and relations, and it lies within each of us. The human organism is the finest observational instrument ever devised
>
> (Deane Juhan, Tulum, Mexico, 1995)

John Cross brings to life the idea of 'listening' to the body through the description of specific 'listening posts' where diagnostic information can be readily obtained. From his long and successful clinical experience, John advises us about when to listen quietly to the phenomena under our fingers, when to listen to our intuition, and when to simply ask the patient what is going on.

For many dedicated therapists, the ideas and experiences which John discusses in this book will make immediate sense and enhance the effectiveness of their hands-on encounters. The information is vital for all who use their hands in the context of healing, even including medical doctors who 'palpate' as a diagnostic procedure, often not realizing the potent effects they may be having on their patients. I am thrilled to see that more and more conventional medical doctors are taking the time to learn specific hands-on techniques such as cranial sacral and acupressure.

John began his explorations with mastery of a discipline and then went on to study other methods, constantly synthesizing, integrating, tinkering, refining, and, beyond all else, paying close attention to the results unfolding under his hands. This is a creative process we all need to engage in, a process by which our comprehension of health and the healing process and of this life within us steadily expands.

Through the various chapters, John takes us along on his exploratory adventure, showing us new possibilities in his clear, direct, personal, and sometimes humorous style. The journey has surprises. For example, he introduces aspects of naturopathic and homeopathic medicine that can enhance our ability to assess a patient and expand the meaning of the information we obtain through physical contact. He takes us into the history of the subject, credits the pioneers, and shows clearly how the concepts relate directly to hands-on work. There is much to be studied here, and John provides abundant and clear illustrations to guide us.

In recent years I have had the opportunity to interact with a wide range of practitioners from many different therapeutic schools, each with a different set of theories and practical techniques. It has been fascinating to see methods evolve toward more effectiveness with less effort on the part of the practitioner. It is also remarkable to see how quickly new ideas such as those you will find in this book can be taken up, explored, and turned into practical applications. Often those skilled in the healing arts turn a new idea into a novel and unanticipated approach. This is an evolutionary collective creative process in action.

I am personally interested in the 'common denominators' underlying all practices, while recognizing that a diversity of approaches is also essential, simply because some patients may respond better to a different type of technique. If you are not connecting with a patient, you can always refer them to another practitioner. But what John Cross and some others are teaching us is the value of having a variety of hands-on methods to hand so that you can shift gears when needed to meet the requirements of your patient.

In this book you will find a wealth of practical common sense information and experience that will benefit any therapist, regardless of background or philosophy. Such a diversity of medical conditions is covered here that this would be a good book to keep in the treatment room to use as a reference for practical day-to-day advice for the general practice situation, whether your patient is presenting with a common cold, chronic back pain, bronchial asthma, depression, or is about to give birth.

Thank you, Dr. Cross, for taking on the monumental effort of communicating your evolutionary process in writing and in illustrations so that all of us can contemplate and benefit. I was thrilled by your first book, and am grateful that you did not stop with that success.

James L. Oschman, PhD
Dover, New Hampshire

Jim Oschman is the author of *Energy Medicine: the scientific basis* (Churchill Livingstone, Edinburgh, 2000) and *Energy Medicine: the therapeutic encounter* (Butterworth Heinemann, Oxford, 2002).

Introduction

This book is the second in a series of books on the subject of acupressure and 'touch' therapies, dedicated to medical professionals. The first in the series, *Acupressure: Clinical Applications in the Treatment of Musculo-skeletal Conditions*, was aimed at the physical therapist who treats chronic spinal and muscular conditions, and has proved to be very successful. It was not meant to represent a complete alternative to all the tried and tested treatments that are carried out in musculo-skeletal conditions, but rather to act as an adjunct to treatment. This book is written along the same lines, in that the author will show the reader many ways to treat medical conditions with touch therapies, in a complementary way to the more orthodox methods. The roots of one's medical training should never be forgotten. There is never just one single answer or approach to a given condition; this book will show a few different ways of treating medical conditions. This book serves as a much-requested sequel, in that it deals with many of the medical conditions that are treated in hospital wards, physical therapy departments and private clinics in everyday practice.

It is important to state that acupressure is *not* a watered down version of acupuncture. There would be very many acupuncturists who would disagree with that statement, insisting that needles have to be 'stuck in' the patient in order to affect energy flow and subsequently get positive results. It is with 25 years' experience of being a successful acupuncture clinician and teacher that I can confidently state that acupressure can be just as effective, as long as it is used correctly and diligently. After all, in traditional Chinese medicine (TCM), 'acupuncture' is a word used to describe *all* aspects of traditional medicine, not just the invasive techniques of needling. Traditional Chinese medicine also includes moxibustion (burning herb), cupping, herbal (internal) medicine, meditation, diet *and* acupressure. There are scores of well-qualified acupuncturists who have almost given up needling to concentrate on acupressure, simply because they achieve better results. Acupressure is also, of course, much more 'patient friendly' and can be used with patients who would prefer not to have needles stuck in them. It can also be used extensively with nervous patients, children and others who prefer touch therapy to invasive therapy.

There are many differences between acupuncture and acupressure, even taking into account that there are many types of acupressure. The main difference, as I see it, is that when using acupressure, the therapist can actually *feel* the various sensations under his or her fingers and hence *know* what is happening within the energy systems of the patient. There is an instant feedback loop that is not always apparent when using acupuncture. In energy balance techniques, the therapist and the patient simultaneously feel the differences in energy quality taking place.

This book also deals with the general philosophy of naturopathy and natural medicine, of which 'touch therapy' represents a small fraction. In my opinion, it is very important not just to use acupressure and touch therapy as a symptomatic 'quick fix', but rather use it as part of a *whole* therapeutic philosophy. When we attempt to help our patients with their various maladies, it is essential that we understand *how* the existing disease within the body has given us certain symptoms and how the patients are externalizing the disease to enable the therapist to make an analysis, assessment or diagnosis. We, as practitioners, do not cure anything – we simply allow the patient to 'heal' themselves by creating a balance where there was imbalance by producing homoeostasis and thus healing. It is the patient's vital force that is utilized, not our own. This is a bedrock statement in any form of natural healing, but it is a message that falls on deaf ears in many quarters.

It has been a pleasure and a privilege to have been asked by Butterworth Heinemann to write this book. They are dedicated to quality dissemination of knowledge to all those involved in the healing and caring professions and have had the foresight to include many aspects of complementary medicine in this goal. I am also delighted that Dr James Oschman has once again written a foreword. It is wonderful to read his words of praise – it is a truly humbling experience.

Finally, I dedicate this book to Andrea, my wife and professional partner of 31 years who has done more than anyone to have been supportive of this and other projects and whose marriage vows of support in sickness and in health have been stretched to the limit over the past few years. Words alone cannot express the love and admiration that I feel for her!

1

Why acupressure?: Vital force: Methods

Why acupressure?

Here you are – a competent therapist, maybe specializing in paediatrics, gynaecology, neurological disease or whatever, being quite happy with your chosen treatment paradigm of exercise therapy, electrotherapy, a little massage and some counselling and obviously doing a good job in your chosen profession. Yet there seems to be something missing! What could it be? This was the way that I was feeling 25 years ago – I was very happy with my treatments and yet I had this desire to be able to do much, much more for my patients – I needed to get more involved with them.

That is why I started to study acupuncture; a bold step indeed for an orthodox therapist in 1975. My peers thought that I was more than a little odd (nothing has changed there) to want to study how to stick needles in people. Comments abounded such as 'Surely it can't work' to 'It must be black magic'. I was a chartered physiotherapist serving with the Royal Marines at the time, so entering the 'weird' world of Chinese medicine was doubly daunting. I practised orthodox physiotherapy during my working day and studied Chinese medicine during the evening and at weekends. It was the beginning of a schizophrenic existence for me that I know that thousands of practitioners have gone through. I left the Royal Marines in 1979 and set up in private practice with my wife and business partner in south Devon. It was there that I learnt that I could not satisfy the needs of my patients or indeed my desire to heal by just concentrating on one philosophy of healing alone. I studied homoeopathy, osteopathy, applied kinesiology, radionics, reflexology, naturopathy and craniosacral therapy and over the years performed all of these, doing what I thought was best for the patient. I am not recommending that every therapist who reads this book embarks on training that is unnecessary – just do that with which you are comfortable. Throughout all of my training, subsequent clinical practice and teaching others, it has been 'hands-on' therapy that has been my greatest love. It probably stems from the fact that my original profession was one of being a chartered physiotherapist, and so I have used my hands for 'healing' since qualifying. It always seemed 'natural' to me to want to 'touch' in order to make others feel well. So, very soon after qualifying as an acupuncturist, I started to combine the two philosophies of physiotherapy and acupuncture – namely acupressure and reflextherapy. I have invented many of my own techniques, some based upon traditional theories, others based upon more modern ones. It has been a great joy for me over the years to be able to teach others these techniques. Many of these are in this book, some were in the last one and there will be many more discussed in the next three.

The question – 'why acupressure?' was asked in the opening title to this chapter. It has still to be answered. This can be done in several ways, but first, the word 'acupressure' needs to be discussed.

What is acupressure?

In the first book, an analogy was made of a Martian landing on earth, asking what acupressure is. The answer to this question was 'energy balancing'. This seems to be a good enough answer to give to someone who does not know the first thing about medicine. Of course there are many different types of acupressure, and these will be discussed later in this chapter, but essentially acupressure is a type of 'hands-on' therapy that attempts to bring about homoeostasis (balance) of energy flow, blood flow, lymphatic, hormonal and nerve conduction. It is a simplistic answer to what is a huge topic. 'Why acupressure' can now be answered.

1. Feeling

As has been mentioned in the Introduction and the early part of this chapter, it is the sensation of being able to *feel* what is happening to the patient as the treatment progresses that is of paramount importance in acupressure. Patients receiving good traditional acupuncture also experience the wonderful (?) sensation of 'de qui' when the needle is correctly inserted. This represents a 'feeling' for the patient and indeed there is a feedback of information between the patient and the therapist because the acupuncturist knows that he or she has hit the acupoint, but there is still no 'feeling' that the practitioner experiences. Naturally, every practitioner is different and not everyone *wants* to 'feel'. Some are quite happy to stay aloof of their patients and simply teach exercises, give electrotherapy or not to get too involved. This in no way is meant as a patronizing remark. Each and every profession has its various facets of approach.

2. Hands on and touch

Clinical acupressure will appeal to those therapists who have entered the 'hands-on' professions, namely physiotherapy, osteopathy, chiropractic, reflexology, massage and kinesiology. It will also appeal to nurses and chiropodists, because they are used to handling people. In my experience, however, it tends not to appeal to those who are wedded to drug therapy, electrotherapy and other forms of 'medicine at a distance'. Each and every person is different and we are all attracted to a particular type of medicine with which we are comfortable. I have taught the art of clinical acupressure to hundreds of students and fellow professionals alike over the years and it has been a privilege to have done so. Not everyone though who has embarked on a course of training has completed the project; some drop out. The dropouts are usually those whose roots are not in other forms of touch therapy, namely doctors, homoeopaths, etc. Also included in this list would be many of the practitioners who are wedded to scientific medicine; this includes acupuncturists who perform only Western scientific acupuncture. Experience has told me that 'touch' can be a very powerful weapon, not everyone can handle it. Also it is ironic that 'touching' has become an anti-social act in the teaching and caring professions. One has to very careful these days, as litigations in malpractice abound. Those of us in the profession though, know how patients long to be 'touched'. Massage is a wonderful way of producing relaxation. When massage is combined with acupressure techniques, the effects on the patient are multiplied. Please, let the profession get back to touching. As was stated in my last book, God gave us hands before He gave us a plug on the wall. Use them!

3. Caring

Acupressure falls under the umbrella of 'caring' professions. It is doubtful whether anyone who enters any branch of medicine does so if they do not have some kind of caring element to their nature. It is essential that anyone who uses clinical acupressure as part of their practice must be able to show empathy with their patients. It seems to me that some therapists and clinicians have lost the ideals of why they entered medicine in the first place. They tend to just go through the motions of treatment and give each patient with similar conditions the same treatment. They have lost sight of the fact that it is the patient that one treats, not necessarily the patient's condition and relevant symptoms. Patients and clients are not numbers, they are human beings. It is a privilege to be able to treat them and we should be honoured that they have chosen us to try and help them. This may seem obvious to some, but it must be stated. The noble art of acupressure is to be taken seriously as a well tried and tested part of natural therapy. It is not to be entered lightly or flippantly or learnt over one or two weekends. It needs commitment and dedication!

4. Non-invasive

This aspect of the therapy is one that is appealing to many practitioners, and is one of the main reasons why they use it. There has been a definite paradigm shift of consciousness over the past two decades (and especially the last 5 years) where invasive medicine has taken a back seat, and the touch therapies, counselling, talking and massage have emerged. Of course, there are some practitioners who prefer to use electrotherapy, needles and the scalpel, but gentle conservative treatments are slowly winning the day. I have noticed particularly that hundreds of acupuncturists now use their hands more and more. It also has to be mentioned that many patients prefer the gentle, non-invasive methods of treatment. Non-invasive therapy is also very good when treating babies, children and people who are nervous or anxious. To be able to touch one's fellow human being in therapy, combined with true empathy and conscientiousness is something that is truly rewarding.

5. Rapport

Of course, it is important that every practitioner has the correct rapport with the patient. Some doctors, nurses and therapists seem to have the bedside manner of a gorilla or a wet slug. It could well be that these people are having a 'bad hair day' and consideration has to be shown in these instances. There is never any excuse, though, to show downright rudeness. Patients are sick human beings and have to have courtesy shown to them. It is with the use of acupressure therapy that rapport with patients really comes into its own. Acupressure is not just a question of twiddling an acupoint and waiting for things to happen – it is usually a question of holding the points and balancing the Chi energy between them. This technique (described later in the chapter) means that one has amazing rapport with the patient. It is not a question of doing and treating, it is a question of harmonizing with the patient to produce an energy balance.

6. Combination of therapies

Very many acupressure therapists use their skills in combination with other therapies or disciplines. It has been mentioned before that the roots of one's medical training should never be forgotten, and one's original skills should be used whenever possible. For instance, it is possible to combine skills as an osteopath and using acupressure in the treatment of musculo-skeletal conditions. It is possible to combine the skills as a reflexologist and using acupressure very easily as the two therapies are intertwined in their theory and practice. It is also possible to combine the skills of acupuncture and using acupressure. The patient could receive acupressure treatment whilst already having the needles *in situ*. It is extremely important that the therapist has a sound knowledge of the subtle body (meridians, reflexes, chakras) to be able to combine the therapies without negating the effect. It is quite true that a patient can be over-treated.

Touch

Touch therapy is one of the oldest forms of treatment in the world, having first been described in China during the second century BCE, then in India, Japan and Egypt. Hippocrates described it as 'the art of rubbing'. During the pharmaceutical revolution of the 1940s, the art of massage sadly declined and physical therapists tended to follow the medical model of 'hands off' approaches. Over the past 10–15 years, however, there has been a tremendous resurgence of 'touch' therapies including massage (in many forms), reflexology, acupressure and shiatsu. Many books have been dedicated to the topic of massage aimed at both the lay person and the medical professional. Hitherto, it was considered that massage was rather 'faddy' and that it was a time-consuming luxury that had no obvious scientific basis. Recently though, many scientific articles and at least two scientifically based books have been published that support its use. This trend is to be welcomed.

Approaches

There are many types and techniques of acupressure that stem basically from three different approaches or philosophies, although there are subdivisions of these three. Although each of these philosophies can stand on its own, and each represents a totality of patient care in its own right, it would be good if they could all be learnt in order to enhance the accuracy of analysis, diagnosis and treatment. The three approaches are traditional oriental (Chinese), traditional Indian (esoteric) touch therapy and reflextherapy. Added to this list would be 'Modern Western' acupressure, based upon the latest physiological knowledge, that uses tender 'trigger' points on the body which are associated with muscles in a state of imbalance. Some of these points bear no similarity to the tried and tested meridian acupoints, some are exactly the same. The author is not experienced in using these symptomatic pain relief points so nothing more will be added on this topic.

Traditional Chinese medicine

Measurement

As today, in the times that traditional Chinese medicine was in its infancy patients were all shapes and sizes – fat and thin, tall or short. Where was the yardstick to provide accurate measurement of where the acupuncture points (acupoints) were? It could not be based on standard units or distance from one point to another using imperial measure. Under the Han Dynasty (202 BCE–220 CE) a solution was found by taking a relative physical measurement, the *cun* (*tchun*) or *pouce*, as the unit of measurement. The patient's own body shape was used, and 1 cun was the width of their thumb at its widest part, which is also equal to the distance between the extent of the skin crease at the distal two joints of the middle finger. Figure 1.1 shows the measurements of the body in terms of cun.

Meridians and vital force

Traditional Chinese medicine (TCM) has been practised for over 5000 years as a way of maintaining health – not necessarily to ease symptoms or to cure. It is believed, though, that acupressure originated in India and later spread to China, Egypt and Asia by Buddhist monks. It is quaintly thought that warriors returning from war exhibiting spear and arrow wounds would be slowly healed of other conditions and disease as their wounds healed, the site of the wound often bearing no relationship to the diseased organ or body part that improved.

Over the years and decades, points were mapped out on the body that had an influence on certain internal organs if they were stimulated. These were called acupoints or *tsubo*. Points on the body that possessed a similar organ affinity were 'joined together' by a series of invisible channels or networks called *meridians*, and each of the meridians was given the name of the organ that it influenced. Names were given to 14 meridians, of which 10 were associated with organs that we understand in orthodox Western medicine, and four others. Two of these 14 are unilateral and 12 are bilateral. There were also an additional six meridians that were mixes and composites of the others, making 20 meridians in all. Acupoints are located

Figure 1.1 The Chinese inch cun measurement.

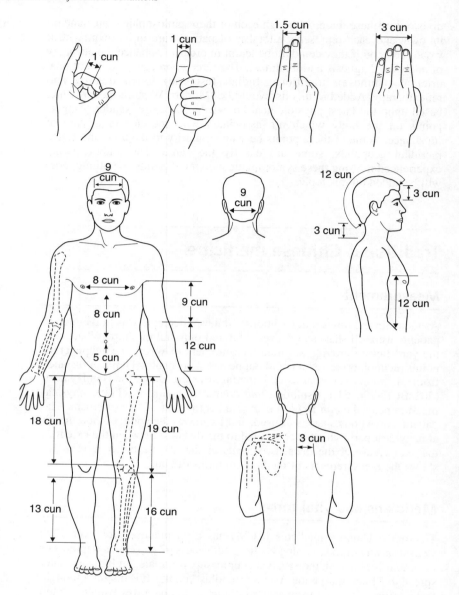

in specific places on the skin and are quite easy to find and detect in that they lie either proximally or distal to certain bony prominences or in hollows made naturally by muscular or tendinous intersections.

Most acupoints are considered to be approximately 1 mm in diameter. When using acupuncture, the needle should pierce the acupoint in order to produce the sensation of *de qui* and to give a better treatment. When using acupressure, the finger and thumb pads are obviously much larger than the acupoint. Treatment is more effective when the acupoint is directly stimulated, but there is an area of influence around each acupoint, especially the important ones, that is anything up to 1 cm away from the point.

The Chinese believed that within the meridians flows an invisible life force energy called *Chi*. It is the manipulation of Chi at the acupoints by stimulation or touch that creates a balance of energy where there was previously an imbalance. In traditional terms, disease=dis-ease=imbalance of energy. The restoration of balance=health. The correlation that is often used with energy flow and the meridian system is to imagine the meridians to be like canals or a waterway system, and the acupoints as lock gates along the canal. When the acupoint is stimulated or touched with intention, the lock gate is opened and the water flows through, energy once more flowing freely through the system. It is said that Chi is an all-pervading and powerful force that exists within every cell in the body. The flow of Chi can best be manipulated at the acupoints, in particular those points between the elbow and fingers and those between the knee and toes. These are called the *command* points. In each meridian there are one or two *great* or influential points that are used more than any other, as experience has shown that they are more effective than others.

From the viewpoint of TCM, there are four components to mention in order to increase the knowledge and awareness of this wonderful form of healing. They are Yin and Yang, the time clock, the law of five elements, and the eight approaches to disease and healing. The time clock was discussed in the last book – it deals with energy flow through the body in the 24-hour cycle. This data will be presented in table form at the beginning of Chapter 3.

Table 1.1 Yin and Yang equivalents

Yang	Yin
Summer	Winter
Heat	Cold
Male	Female
Light	Dark
Acute	Chronic
Spastic	Flaccid
Mobility	Stiffness
Inflammation	Oedema
Hypertension	Hypotension
Hollow organs	Vital organs
Heaven	Earth
Energy/Thought	Matter/Substance
Expansion	Contraction
Extrovert	Introvert
Aggressive	Passive
Fast	Slow

Yin and Yang

These two words (properly pronounced 'inn' and 'arng') represent the two bi-polars of Chi, and are opposite and yet complementary to each other. They will be mentioned time and time again in this book. They form the backbone of thought in many of the traditional and ancient medical philosophies. Some authorities believe that a deep knowledge of the bi-polar energy forces of Yin and Yang may explain many aspects of the cosmos itself as well as the workings of the human body. In simple terms, Yang covers the acute side of disease and Yin covers the chronic. Table 1.1 gives a few Yin and Yang equivalents.

Figure 1.2 shows the symbol known as the *pakua* or the Chinese monad. The roundness indicates wholeness, which, according to the Chinese, is simply called Chi. The shaded area is Yin and the light area is Yang. Please note that the division is not a straight line but a curved one – nothing in nature or the human body is straight; nothing is black and white but all is various shades of grey. Note also that there is a little Yin in the Yang and a little Yang in the Yin. Put in therapy terms, there are never wholly Yin or Yang conditions. Total Yin is, of course, death of the physical body. Generally speaking, where there is a predominantly Yang condition there is pain, inflammation, heat and redness, and this condition needs to be sedated in order to balance the energy. Where there is a predominantly Yin condition there could also be pain, but the area may be stiff, chronic, sluggish or oedematous etc. and this needs to be stimulated in order to balance the Chi. There is a golden rule in medicine that the acute needs to be addressed firstly before the chronic nature of the dis-ease can be unravelled and treated. In acupressure, the same point can be used to stimulate or sedate, depending on the way it is treated, hence giving a

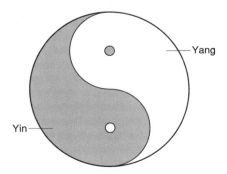

Figure 1.2 The Chinese monad.

different sensation and result. The meridians may also be placed in a Yin/Yang context as follows:

Yang	Yin
Small intestine	Heart
Bladder	Kidney
Large intestine	Lung
Gall bladder	Liver
Stomach	Spleen
Three heater	Pericardium
Governor	Conception

It is important that these are memorized as Yin/Yang couples. The latter two pairs will be explained later. Note that the Yang organs are hollow, peristaltic in nature and not vital to life, whereas the Yin organs are solid ones that are essential to life. It is obvious with all the surgical advances recently that people can live without the spleen or one kidney, but it has to be remembered that these organs and subsequent energy channels control more than Western medicine appreciates. The spleen, for instance, is said to be the home of the immune system, and has important uses in gynaecological conditions.

The law of five elements (transformations)

This law was explained in the last book, but it probably holds more significance in the treatment of medical conditions than in the treatment of musculo-skeletal conditions. Each organ is placed in one of five 'elements', the Yang organs being on the outside (representing 'superficial') and the Yin on the inside (representing 'deep'), with the Yin/Yang couples opposite each other (Figure 1.3). The *Sheng* or engendering cycle is said to be the creative cycle, and the *Ko* cycle is said to be the controlling cycle. The five elements are not chemical elements but rather five aspects of the world, nature and the human frame that represent the rhythms of life.

In the Sheng cycle, fire produces ashes (earth); earth (as ore) produces metal; metal (by hydrolysis) produces water; water produces wood in the sense that water makes plant life possible; wood produces fire as in fuel.

In the Ko cycle, fire subjugates metal as in melting; metal subjugates wood as in chopping or cutting; wood subjugates earth by penetrating it with roots; earth subjugates water by absorbing it or providing a dam or obstruction; water subjugates fire by extinguishing it. Table 1.2 represents a fraction of the many and various aspects of this law and shows what can be placed into each element.

Examples of clinical importance

1. Patients can sometimes be archetyped according to which system and part of the body is affected. With this knowledge, the therapist can treat the relevant meridian and acupoints. For example, a person who suffers from irritable bowel syndrome, has a pale skin, suffers from catarrh, feels worse in the autumn and in dry weather would be placed as a 'metal' person. The archetyping is not usually as clear-cut as the example given but it is also rare that just one single element energy

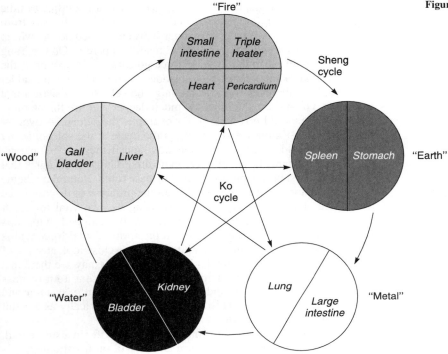

Figure 1.3 The law of five elements.

imbalance needs to be addressed. There is a 'batting' order of treatment that will be explained in Chapter 4.

2. Chi energy can be transferred from element to element, thus providing a balance of energy within the body. This is a very good way in which to finish a treatment session. This procedure is covered in Chapter 5.

3. By taking a correct case history, the therapist will be able to ascertain how condition has followed condition, seemingly at random but actually always in a logical plan according to the Ko cycle. As stated before, disease can be likened to that of an energy force, being opposite to vital force. Whereas vital force is always engendering and health improving, so disease force works in the opposite way. Once

Table 1.2 The law of five elements

	Fire	*Earth*	*Metal*	*Water*	*Wood*
Direction	South	–	West	North	East
Colour	Red	Yellow	White	Black	Green
System	Circulation	Connective tissue	Skin	Bones	Muscles, tendons
Face	Tongue	Mouth	Nose	Ears	Eyes
Emotion	Excess joy	Depression	Grief	Fear	Anger
Season	Summer	Late summer	Autumn (fall)	Winter	Spring
Taste	Bitter	Sweet	Pungent	Salt	Sour
Weather	Heat	Humidity	Dryness	Cold	Wind
Sense	Speech	Taste	Smell	Hearing	Sight

dis-ease has entered the body by whatever way that is outlined in the next chapter, disease force or destructive force rampages its way from organ to organ in a 'reverse Ko' manner. This quite often occurs within the Yang organs when illness is not so readily apparent. On the Yang cycle this would mean that disease force goes from, for example, the large intestine → small intestine → bladder → stomach → gall bladder and completes the cycle back at the large bowel. Once disease force enters the Yin system, the illness is much deeper and life threatening. Disease force would travel from, for example, the spleen → liver → lung → heart → kidney and completes the cycle at the spleen. Many treatments would be tried along the way, and if they are allopathic, they would probably be suppressive in nature. Many experts agree that this actually hastens the progression of disease force. Natural medicine (of which acupressure is one) would halt the progress of disease force and would enable the body to fight by using its own vital force. Of course, the human body is extremely well equipped with this superhuman self-healing mechanism in the form of vital force and is therefore always attempting to heal itself. Take a close look at some of your patients with their particular histories and you may see them in a new light. The law of five elements does not represent a hit or miss philosophy of 'let's try this and see what *may* happen', it *is* a *law* and as such is always correct. This is stated quite categorically as a result of 25 years of experience in traditional medicine.

4. Take, for example, the case of someone who has suffered a stroke with resultant painful spasticity of an arm and leg. If, on questioning, it is found that the pain and discomfort are worse for being hot and definitely worse in the summer, that they have problems with their speech, have a bitter taste in the mouth and have a rather ruddy complexion, the practitioner can deduce that they are a 'Fire' person. This means that the Fire element organ/meridians of three heater, small intestine, heart and pericardium need to be stimulated (usually at the source point) together with the 'mother' of the Fire, namely the 'Wood' meridians of gall bladder and liver. It is useless to give localized therapy symptomatically if the general Chi energy has not been addressed.

It can be seen from just giving the few examples above how complicated this law actually is, but how fascinating a study it also is. Scholars have struggled with the ramifications of this law over a lifetime and still not fully explored it.

The eight approaches

The traditional Chinese doctor (or barefoot doctor, as they were known) would make a thorough and comprehensive examination of the patient by firstly taking a case history. He would then observe and listen to the patient, then touch and palpate the symptomatic areas, look at the tongue, look at the eyes and palpate the abdomen. The findings of this clinical examination would be placed under the eight key symptoms or approaches of TCM, namely Deep and Superficial; Cold and Heat; Emptiness and Fullness and finally Yin and Yang. These differentials enabled the doctor to ascertain the energetic imbalance and to determine the severity of the ailment. Emptiness indicates an energy deficiency and includes such symptoms as lack of appetite, night sweats and lassitude. Fullness indicates an acute disorder and includes symptoms such as excess phlegm, flatulence and constipation. If the patient does not feel thirsty or prefers hot drinks there is a Cold condition, whereas thirst for cold drinks, dry lips, red eyes and general listlessness are symptoms of Heat. Pains in the peripheral joints are called Superficial, and pains in the chest and abdomen are called Deep. Yin and Yang are the basic principles for the functioning of the whole organism and also the others: hence Yang can cover Superficial, Heat and Fullness, and Yin can cover Cold, Deep and Emptiness. Quite often, as in Western medicine, the object of the treatment is to convert a chronic condition into an acute one in order to make it easier to treat; thus we attempt to turn Cold into Heat, Deep into Superficial, Emptiness into Fullness and Yin into Yang.

Traditional Japanese medicine (TJM) is very similar to TCM. Probably the best known aspect of it is the art of shiatsu. Shiatsu is a Japanese word made up of two written characters meaning finger (*shi*) and pressure (*atsu*). The acupuncture points used in shiatsu are called *tsubo*, and treatment consists of pressure on these and broad areas using fingers, thumbs, elbows and sometimes feet. More details about TJM are to be found in the book on musculo-skeletal conditions. Suffice it to say, although shiatsu is a total treatment concept and can be very effective in its own right, it does *not* represent the whole of the acupressure umbrella, contrary to popular belief.

Traditional Indian (esoteric) touch therapy

It is said that the human frame consists of an interpenetrating series of body forms of different frequency vibrations, ranging from the physical to the spiritual, with the higher spiritual and mental frequency forms determining the state of the physical body. The appreciation of the existence of the subtle bodies is the bedrock of the understanding of subtle body healing. The *chakras* are considered to be force centres or whorls of energy situated at particular points on the physical body and permeating through the layers of the other subtle bodies in an ever-increasing fan-shaped formation. They are rotating vortices of subtle matter, and are considered to be the focal points for the transmission and reception of energies. Up until recently, use of the *chakras* and the other higher centres of energy have been reserved for the traditional Eastern medicines and religions and in the practice of yoga and meditation. Information from various ancient texts of Indian yogic literature give mention to these special force centres or chakras that exist on the surface of the body, having internal relationships and associations (including nerve plexuses and endocrine glands) and yet having a more subtle, and more powerful, association with our bodies and aura, The word *chakra* means 'wheel' in Sanskrit. Each chakra has particular landmarks, and each is represented by a different vibrational rate, colour, endocrine gland, nerve plexus and set of symptoms should any imbalance occur. There are said to be seven major chakras and 21 minor chakras. The minor chakras are said to be reflected points of the majors and do not extend any further than the etheric body outwards. Each point, though, is considered to be a very powerful acupoint, equivalent to a 'great' point. The positioning of the chakras will

Table 1.3 Some associations of the major chakras

Chakra	Coupled minors	Endocrine	Organ	Meridian(s)	Acupoints
1. Crown	Hand and Foot	Pineal	Upper brain, right eye	Triple heater	Gov 20
2. Brow	Clavicular and Groin	Pituitary	Nervous system, ears, nose, left eye	Gall bladder	Gov 16, Yintang
3. Throat	Shoulder and Navel	Thyroid	Bronchial, lungs, large bowel	Large intestine and lung	Gov 14, Con 22
4. Heart	Ear and Intercostal	Thymus	Heart, circulation, vagus nerve	Heart and small intestine	Gov 10, Con 17
5. Solar plexus	Spleen	Pancreas	Stomach, liver, spleen, pancreas	Liver and stomach	Gov 6, Con 14
6. Sacral	Spleen	Gonads	Reproductive system, fluid balance	Spleen and pericardium	Gov 3, Con 6
7. Base	Elbow and Knee	Adrenals	Spinal column, kidney, bladder	Bladder and kidney	Gov 2, Con 2

be shown in Chapter 3 but Tables 1.3 and 1.4 show their relationships and associations.

There are said to be 21 minor chakras, which are reflected points of the majors. There are 10 bilateral minor chakras plus the spleen, which some authorities consider to be equal to a major chakra in its power and influence.

It has been my onerous but pleasant task over the past 20 years to attempt to explain the chakra energy system in Western orthodox terms and attempt to de-mystify it. For more details of this system please refer to my chapter in *Complementary Therapies for Physical Therapists* published by Butterworth Heinemann. Also, a book on the subject is being planned.

Table 1.4 Associations of the minor chakras

Minor chakra	Coupled minor	Coupled major	Acupoint
Foot	Hand	Crown	Ki 1
Hand	Foot	Crown	P 8
Knee	Elbow	Base	Bl 40
Elbow	Knee	Base	P 3
Groin	Clavicular	Brow	St 30
Clavicular	Groin	Brow	Ki 27
Shoulder	Navel	Throat	LI 15
Navel	Shoulder	Throat	Ki 16
Intercostal	Ear	Heart	Sp 21
Ear	Intercostal	Heart	TH 17
Spleen	–	Solar plexus and Sacral	Sp 16 right

Reflextherapy

The use and practice of foot reflexology has lasted as long as acupuncture and acupressure and has its roots firmly entrenched in traditional oriental medicine, but the modern practice of 'zone therapy' began with an American specialist, Dr William Fitzgerald. Dr Fitzgerald noticed that his patients varied in the amount of pain that they suffered in the post-operative state. He discovered that his patients who had performed their own kind of 'painful point therapy' on the feet faired better than those patients who were ignorant of such procedures. He researched at length into this and discovered that the body can be divided into 10 equal sections (five on each side of the body) along its vertical plane from head to feet. These sections were not just on the skin but appeared to affect underlying organs as well. An American masseuse, Eunice Ingham, was interested in Dr Fitzgerald's work and she concentrated her efforts in mapping out both vertical and horizontal zones on the feet, as well as body points. She invented what is a major philosophy of reflexology, namely foot zonal therapy. In the beginning, this therapy concentrated on the joints, mainly of the hands and feet, with the use of heavy pressure lasting up to a few minutes in duration. This type of reflextherapy has since evolved to become the most popular form used in the Western world. Figure 1.4 shows the horizontal and vertical reflexes of the feet.

Figure 1.4 Vertical and horizontal reflexes.

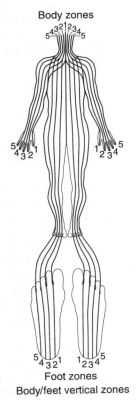

Body zones

Foot zones
Body/feet vertical zones

Level of reflexes on the feet

Types of reflextherapy

Since the original foot zonal therapy, other forms of reflextherapy have emerged. Some of them encompass zone therapy as their basis, but others use the Chinese meridian system, the organic system, the organic-joint system and some use the reflex energy centres. Each of the types assumes that the whole of the body can be mapped on the feet, this giving a microcosm within the macrocosm. Types of reflexology include: 'foot reflexology', 'vertical reflextherapy', 'precision reflextherapy', 'reflexology with meridian therapy', 'organic reflexology', 'universal reflexology', 'zone therapy' and 'light touch reflexology'. The amount of pressure that is used by the therapist on his or her patient/client depends upon the type of reflexology that has been studied and practised. This ranges from using extremely heavy massage on tender points to hardly touching at all. So, there appears to be a mish-mash of ideas and approaches to this wonderful form of healing. It will always remain the case that the practitioner will perform the type of 'hands-on' therapy that is comfortable for him or her and the one with which they achieve the best results. It is 'horses for courses'. Charts showing the foot reflexes that are used in acupressure are shown in Chapter 2.

There are, of course, many other areas of the body, apart from the feet, where reflexes appear. It is considered that there are as many as 14 areas of reflexes (or reflected areas) on the body that can be used for diagnostic purposes and 10 reflected areas that may be used for treatment. The diagnostic areas are the iris, tongue, teeth, face, temple, pulse, hand, skull (three types), ear, foot, abdomen (two types), spine (several types) as well as major and minor chakras and meridians. There are also the so-called 'listening posts'. The areas that can be used in treatment are on the ear, skull, temple, face, hands, feet, abdomen, spine, chakras and meridians. Many reflexologists have the impression that reflex points only appear on the hands and feet. Nothing is further from the truth.

Symptomatic and holistic

It has previously been mentioned that there are many approaches to reflextherapy, but each can be broadly placed into one of two categories – symptomatic and holistic. In many types of symptomatic reflextherapy, the reflected points and pathways of the organ or body part that is 'sick' is treated by several 'touch' methods. These techniques are often very effective and are sometimes exactly what is required by the patient. A whole reflexology treatment of, say, an hour's duration will consist of the symptomatic treatment of many of the organ and body systems, each one flowing into the next one. The effect of such treatment is to give relaxation to the affected parts, thus allowing self-healing to take place – at least that *should* be the maxim of the practitioner. With the holistic approaches to reflextherapy and acupressure that are discussed in this book, the symptoms are used by the therapist as merely a guide to eventually arrive at the true *cause* of the imbalance. During the case history and subsequent initial feel of the feet (see next chapter) the holistic practitioner should always have regard to the cause of the problem. It is imperative that a thorough case history is taken that includes physical symptoms past and present, weaknesses or strengths of certain areas of the body, emotional and mental history, effects of old viral infections etc., etc. It is by treating the cause of the dis-ease by energy balancing that allows a much deeper and effective treatment to take place. The therapist will find that fewer treatment sessions are required and that the results are gained more rapidly.

Reflexes

What is a reflex? When this question is asked of delegates at the start of a workshop, heads lower! Each delegate assumes that someone else will come up with a brilliant answer. Could it be a trick question? What is he getting at? It is not a trick question at all! Some would consider a reflex to be a nerve ending on the foot, others would say that it is a crystalline deposit of uric acid and calcium that builds up on the foot when an organ is congested. Yet others would say that a reflex is part of the meridian system as used in acupuncture. In his book *Reflex Zone Massage*, Franz Wagner* suggests that we could think of the body as a hologram and that within this hologram, each of the millions of cells would be further holograms. Each cell would carry the basic information about all the other cells and about the whole body. This explanation is to be applauded and is very close to my own philosophy. A reflex is an abbreviation of the word *reflected*. A reflex is therefore a *reflected* point or pathway that appears on the several areas of the body already mentioned. By its very nature, it falls into the realm of 'energy' medicine which purports to use 'vital force'. If the reflexes on the body can be considered as just that – reflected points of energy – then it follows that there is an energetic link between the part of the body that is undergoing a state of imbalance or disharmony, and its reflected point. It further means that by simple light touch on the reflected point, the practitioner can affect the flow of energy to the part of the body that has the imbalance. Such an explanation would also adequately describe an acupoint. The reflex or acupoint does *not* have to be beaten into submission by harsh and heavy massage, however much the patient may feel that it is doing them good. Many patients are conditioned into the mode of thought of 'no pain – no gain' (as are some practitioners).

Methods of treatment

The most common techniques of hands-on healing are performed with the tips and pads of the fingers and thumbs, with some use of the hands as a whole and occasionally the ulnar border of the hand or even the elbow. There are six different ways of affecting the energy flow in an acupuncture point, meridian or area of the body:

1. Light touch on a point.
2. Deep touch on a point.
3. Gentle massage on a point.
4. Stimulating massage on a point.
5. Light massage on an area or meridian.
6. Stimulating massage on an area or meridian.

*Wagner, Franz. *Reflex Zone Massage* (1987) Thorsons.

Light touch on a point

This is performed either with the forefinger or the middle finger pad, and is simply the placing of the finger on a point with hardly any pressure and with no other part of the hand in contact with the patient. The actual fingers that are used are very important, and this will be discussed later on in the chapter.

Uses:

1. To transfer energy from a point or an area to another point or area. By touching various powerful acupoints and reflex points, the energetic quality of internal organs or other areas of the body can be affected.
2. To draw away excess Yang (heat and inflammation) from a distal point or area.
3. To balance energy between two points. This can either be performed on two points of the same meridian to effect a natural flow of Chi or between a proximal point and distal point of differing meridians. In this case, the distal point is called a Great point.

Deep touch on a point

This technique can be performed with a single finger pad or with the fore-, middle or ring fingers in close proximity if there are adjacent acupoints to be treated. The fingers are placed on the acupoint or reflex point, very gently at first (always having regard for the patient's tissues, energy and aura) and progressively getting deeper and deeper into the tissues and working up to the patient's tolerance. This technique should *never* be painful or uncomfortable, and the pressure used should be tolerable and performed very slowly to accommodate the patient's pain threshold and comfort.

Uses:

1. In local inflammatory (Yang) areas, where the excess energy has to be dispersed either by placing just one finger on the area or by balancing that point with another point.
2. To release muscle spasm and tension in the tissues and thus bring about harmony in the circulation (blood and lymphatics). Essentially, this technique of acupressure is for localized inflammatory areas where excess heat and inflammation need to be released. The therapist, with experience, may hold the point for up to 5 minutes whilst his or her fingers get progressively warmer. It is a technique that is very rewarding for the patient in the relief of pain. The therapist should never be in a hurry to somehow force the movement of energy and thus establish a harmony. Never *will* things to happen – let them happen by themselves. Generally, the more chronic the condition, the longer it takes to treat.

Gentle massage on a point

This is performed with the finger or thumb pads, and should be very gentle with no stimulation at all.

Uses:

1. To calm a patient, using certain acupoints prior to the main treatment.
2. To treat sub-acute conditions where the underlying condition is chronic (Yin), but superficially it is essentially painful and inflamed (Yang).
3. In reflexology, this gentle form of massage may be performed on the feet and hand reflexes. Reflex points and many acupoints are reflected pathways of other points of energy, and should not be 'blasted' with stimulating massage. Much more positive results will be obtained by using gentle massage than by digging the thumbs in and trying to bore a hole in the patient's tissues.

Gentle massage on a point should not be performed in any condition where there is a localized disease area, e.g. growth, tumour, internal organ infection, rheumatoid joint etc. Disease can be likened to a force that can easily be spread (see next chapter). Conditions such as rheumatoid arthritis can be helped with acupressure, but never use stimulating massage. *Never, never, never* perform any stimulating massage in neurological conditions such as multiple sclerosis.

Stimulating massage on a point

This technique is very similar to circular frictions as used in the treatment of soft tissue injuries and sports injuries (how physiotherapists love these!). It is to be used *only* where there is a chronic or underlying chronic condition, and where energy needs to be created or stimulated. As well as using the finger and thumb pads, it can also be performed with the ulnar border of the hand at the pisiform bone, or with the elbow when it is used on the spine. This is popular in shiatsu.

Uses:

1. Treating localized chronic (Yin) conditions where the area needs stimulation of energy via the acupoints, e.g. chronic tennis elbow or the local symptoms of frozen shoulder.
2. To stimulate the flow of energy down a meridian where there is chronic pain and discomfort at the distal end of the meridian, e.g. massaging LI 4 for chronic sinusitis.
3. To stimulate the flow of lymphatic drainage by massaging the so called neuro-lymphatic points or Chapman's reflexes. As previously mentioned, stimulating massage should not be performed on foot and hand reflexes (contrary to the popularly taught theories of zone therapy) in cases of neurological or central nervous system conditions. It is also contraindicated during the first 3 months of pregnancy and at menstruation.

Light massage on an area or meridian

This is performed with either the fingertips or the hand as a whole, and is simply the brushing of the skin with the gentlest of touches – no stimulation whatsoever. Because of its subtlety, there is no need to even touch the actual skin, and often patients may keep their clothes on.

Uses:

1. On a meridian from the entry of the meridian to its exit, i.e. from the Tsing (end) point to the last point or vice versa, depending on whether energy in the meridian as a whole needs to be simulated or sedated. Massage with the flow of energy to stimulate energy in the meridian and against the flow of energy to sedate or lessen the energy flow.
2. When an area of the body is being prepared for more specific work at a later stage of treatment. This would constitute effleurage in orthodox massage.
3. In a diagnostic way when an area is palpated to ascertain certain underlying structural or soft tissue anomalies, e.g. abdominal diagnosis (see Chapter 2).

Stimulating massage on an area or meridian

This is performed with a finger or thumb pad or with the inner border of the middle finger, and is essentially used as a stimulating massage in chronic (Yin) illness. It is used when a meridian or part of a meridian needs to be stimulated in order to bring more energy to the area or underlying organ connection. An example of this would be thumb pad kneading along the course of the bladder meridian in chronic lower spinal conditions or cystitis. This technique of acupressure stimulates the stagnation of Chi energy due to a build up of fatty deposits, scar tissue, fibrous tissue or cellulite. The whole length of the meridian need not be massaged, but as much as is practicable gives better results. This massage does not necessarily have to be performed with the flow of energy, but results will be improved if it is. Another example of using this technique is stimulating massage along the course of the large intestine and lung meridians in the treatment of chronic catarrh.

Types of acupressure

There are several types of clinical acupressure that can be used in the treatment of medical conditions. Those that are performed using the meridian system of energy are the use of local points, distal points, local and distal points, parallel points, great points, associated effect points, specific points and meridian massage. Other types of acupressure that utilize non-meridian energy flow include ear, scalp, abdominal, hand and foot acupressure (reflextherapy) and by using the major and minor chakras.

Local points

These points are local to the inflammatory (Yang) or chronic (Yin) part of the body that is being treated, e.g. LI 20 in the treatment of sinusitis or GB 20 in the treatment of occipital headache. The technique and pressure that the therapist uses depends on the underlying condition and 'feel' of the tissues. In obvious acute conditions where there is heat, inflammation and some localized swelling, the finger(s) is/are gently placed on the points, *slowly* getting deeper and deeper into the tissues (to the patient's tolerance of discomfort) until heat is liberated in the area. There is sometimes a need to hold such a point for up to 10 minutes or until the majority of the 'heat' is dispersed. Local point acupressure though is not so common in medical condition treatment as it is in musculo-skeletal conditions. In sub-acute conditions, albeit with a superficial inflammatory state (such as in rheumatoid arthritis), the fingers are placed as before and, when all the heat has been subdued, gentle circular massage is performed on the point in order to stimulate the underlying Yin condition. In chronic conditions (which will probably cover most of the average therapy workload), the local points are first gently stimulated with circular finger-pad massage, followed by more robust massage on the same point. In *all* chronic (Yin) conditions, energy needs to be summoned (stimulated) in order to be used. A 'reservoir' of energy needs to be created. The golden rule in acupressure is to *sedate* the Yang (acute) and *stimulate* the Yin (chronic).

Distal points

This type of acupressure deals with affecting energy at a distance on a meridian that lies local to the condition but where localized treatment is impossible to do, such as with open wounds, or underlying pathology. The underlying meridian must be known, as treatment will be focused either on the Tsing (end) point or another point of great influence at the distal end of the meridian. Where the underlying condition is acute, the distal point should just be held until the heat and pain eases from the local area. In sub-acute conditions, gentle massage should be used on the point and stimulating massage should be used in the case of chronic conditions. Examples of using distal acupressure include the use of Bl 67 and St 45 in acute conjunctivitis, and the use of LI 4 and LI 1 in acute toothache. Other types of distal acupressure use the reflected areas (reflexes) already mentioned. Each and every part of the body has a number of associated (or reflected) points and areas, and there is usually a plethora of choice. Because there is a direct link with the organ, the distal point (acupoint or reflex) just needs to be held gently for about 2 minutes until there is a change of energy emphasis and healing and energy flow commences. In the cases of chronic and sub-acute conditions, the distal point needs mild stimulation for about half a minute prior to holding the point.

Local and distal points

The use of local and distal points together is the most common type of acupressure that is used by therapists. Although with single point acupressure there is a certain amount of feel and change of awareness under the finger, it is with the combined local and distal points that the awareness of energy movement is most demonstrated. It is possible, with practice, to be able to feel the flow of energy taking place. What is more, patients often feel changes too – after all, it is their energy system that is being affected. Patients who are used to acupressure treatment will often inform the therapist that a change in sensation has occurred before the therapist feels it. The sensations that can occur were discussed fully in the last book. They include heat, pulsing, tingling, cold and buzzing. The overall sensation that is felt though, after a couple minutes of holding the points is one of *harmony* or one-ness with the patient. This sensation will be discussed later in the book, but for now, please remember that with this type of acupressure, the therapist is *balancing* energy between two points – nothing more, nothing less. They are *not* imparting any of their own energy or taking part in any mystical 'healing'. There are several ways of performing local and distal acupressure:

1. Balancing points that are on the same meridian.
2. Balancing points using the local point and a Great point that is not on the same meridian as the distal point.
3. Balancing points using the local point and a major reflex point (foot, hand, ear, scalp).
4. Balancing points using the local point and the nearest chakra point.
5. Balancing points that lie on the same zone of energy.
6. Balancing points using the local point and its parallel point.

The rationale of balancing energy in reflexes is the same as balancing energy using local and distal points on the same meridian. (That statement would appear to be blasphemous in some quarters!)

1. Balancing points on the same meridian

With each of the methods of energy balancing described below, it is essential that the therapist is comfortable with the arms supported as much as possible. Points may be held sometimes for up to 10 minutes! Once the two points are correctly found, gentle stimulation of the points should take place for a few seconds. This helps to reinforce the energy potential within the meridian, even if the condition is acute. For the remainder of the technique, the fingers are placed gently onto the skin, with no pressure whatsoever, waiting for the change of energy emphasis to take place. Once this has occurred, the points may be held for as long as you like, but 2 minutes is adequate to achieve a balance of energy. In the case of very long-standing chronic conditions, the energy needs to summoned. In this case, the two points need to be stimulated for about half a minute. This does not mean that a hole is bored into the tissues. Experience will tell when it is time to change from the stimulation to the holding. There will be an alteration of feel of the tissues under the fingers, in that they will appear to be more pliable and warmer.

Example of balancing points on the same meridian – acute stomach pain (gastritis)

The points used are Con 14 and Con 6. The therapist places the middle finger of either hand on point Con 14 (this is the point on the conception meridian that is nearest anatomically to the stomach) and touches gently for a few seconds so that the patient gets used to the feel. The middle finger of the other hand is then introduced on to Con 6 and the therapist holds the two points for a few seconds. Initially there will be a difference in feel under the two points. As the two points are held, a similarity in feeling will be felt. This can either be the same type of pulsing, heat, buzzing etc., but essentially it has to be the *same* sensation. When the same sensation is felt the patient should find that the discomfort has either gone or changed after a couple of minutes. When the fingers are held *in situ* longer than the time taken to achieve a balance of energy between the two points, a 'change in emphasis' will occur. As mentioned elsewhere, this sensation occurs when the 'alpha–theta' brainwave frequency is reached and both patient and therapist are in 'harmony' (see Figure 1.5).

2. Balancing energy between the local point and a Great point

This is performed in exactly the same way as the previous example. The difference being that the distal point has more available energy to hand, so the procedure is more effective and takes less time to complete the procedure. Great points are those acupoints on the body that have more energy influence and are used for more than one purpose (explained later in Chapter 3).

Example of balancing points using a great point – acute stomach pain

The points used are Con 14 (as before) and St 36. The symptom of stomach pain is purposely used again as an example in order to illustrate how the same condition may be treated using two different approaches. This is also a way of stressing that there are no hard and fast rules when it comes to healing with acupressure. St 36 is an extremely important point that is used for many conditions associated with the stomach, pain in the abdomen and general lethargy. The same procedure is carried out as before, with the exception that St 36 will need more gentle stimulation than a point that lies on the same meridian. The therapist will note that, when using these points, a balance of energy will be effected quite quickly, but this

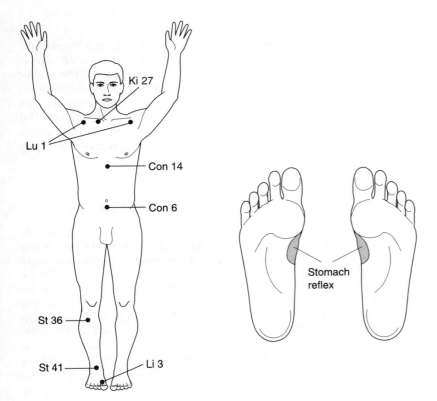

Figure 1.5 Examples of local and distal point acupressure.

does not necessarily help the pain. The reason for this is that 'pain' is a complex issue and has come about because of the patient's complex physiological changes; therefore it is not always possible to ease deep-seated pain immediately (see Figure 1.5).

3. Balancing energy between the local point and a reflex point

As explained before, my personal view is that there is no difference between an acupoint and a reflex when used in practice. The technique therefore is exactly the same as the previous two. One finger is placed on the local point and the corresponding reflex point is balanced with the same finger of the other hand. Details of the exact fingers used are detailed at the end of this chapter. When attempting to find the distal reflex point, it is necessary that not too much pressure and 'feeling around' is done, so as not to make the patient too sore. The exact reflex correspondence will exhibit tenderness when felt. It is sufficient to gently stimulate the local point and reflex point for a few seconds before the two points are held, as before, until a shift of emphasis occurs. The shift is not quite so apparent or obvious as with the other two, but it does occur, so patience is required. This particular technique is from the branch of reflextherapy called 'light touch reflexology'. When using the reflex point, the other point to be balanced does not have to be a local point that is close to a 'lesion'. It could be any other point that is associated with the reflex.

Example of balancing energy between an acupoint and a reflex point – stomach pain

The points used are St 36 (previously described) and the tender part of the stomach reflex on the foot. The same condition is purposely used so as to again demonstrate the versatility of acupressure techniques. The middle finger of one hand is placed gently on St 36 and the middle finger of the other hand is placed on the stomach reflex. Make sure that the forearms are well supported as this hold could be for up to 10 minutes in duration. This technique is often the most effective of all the ones described in this section and would probably be the preferential choice of reflexologists (see Figure 1.5).

4. Balancing energy between the acupoint and the nearest chakra point

Using the same example of stomach pain, the acupoint used could be any one on the stomach meridian that has an affinity for pain relief. Although St 36 is an effective and much used point, the example here will use St 41. This point is situated on the midpoint of the dorsum of the foot at the ankle crease, between the tendons of extensor digitorum and halucis longus. It is a very easy point to find. The corresponding chakra point would be the acupoint correspondence of the solar plexus chakra, which is the chakra that deals with digestion. This point is Con 14 which is situated at the base of the xiphoid process in the midline. The practitioner will find that the energy balance in this case will occur twice as quickly as the others (see Figure 1.5).

5. Balancing energy between two points lying on the same zone

If the same example of stomach pain is used, the fingers of each hand may be placed on any influential point proximal and distal to the area of pain, as long as they all lie on the same vertical zone. Imagine that the pain is in the part of the stomach that lies in Zone 2, the proximal point could be Ki 27 and the distal point could be St 25. If the therapist does not produce an energy balance after holding the points for about 2 minutes, then the fingers are in the wrong place! Of all the ways of balancing energy, this seems to be the most unsatisfactory in terms of effectiveness and satisfaction – but it still works! (see Figure 1.5).

6. Balancing between parallel points

Parallel point acupressure is the use of the same point on the opposite limb. It is used when it is impossible to do local point acupressure, e.g. gravitational ulcer, or it can be used as an adjunct to other forms of acupressure. It seems to be highly effective in certain conditions. When there is a discontinuity of the skin (ulceration) or a burn etc. and it is therefore impossible to place the fingers locally, the *exact* point on the opposite limb is used. Using the example of treating the pain of a gravitational ulcer which occurs around the lower two-thirds of the medial aspect of the tibia and is quite often centred on point Sp 6, the treatment is to stimulate the opposite Sp 6 for anything up to 5 minutes. Other points may be stimulated as long as they are parallel to the acute or chronic inflammation. They do not necessarily have to be meridian points, but if they are on a meridian it will enhance the treatment.

Parallel point acupressure can also be used as an adjunct to other types of acupressure. For instance, in the case of an acutely painful chest condition, as well as performing local and distal acupressure along the conception meridian or between Lu 1 and Lu 7, the two Lu 1 points may be gently stimulated and held. This can be for anything up to 10 minutes. Some amazing results can be obtained with this procedure (see Figure 1.5).

Meridian massage

This can be used for both stimulation and sedation.

Stimulation

This is performed with the finger pad or thumb pad kneading along the meridian and is done in the direction of energy flow, i.e. from the Tsing point to the end point. This stimulates the energy flow and is useful in underlying chronic conditions, e.g. thumb pad kneading along the course of the lung and large intestine meridians would be useful in the treatment of chronic respiratory and skin conditions. It is a very helpful technique with which to commence most treatments dealing with chronic conditions. It also eases stagnation of Chi along the course of a channel (meridian) due to fatty deposits, cellulite or fibrositic nodules. The whole length of the meridian need not be massaged. A stimulating type of massage can also be performed using the whole hand and stroking along the meridian in the direction of energy flow. It can even be done through thin clothing, and can be quite effective in the initial stimulation of energy in the particular meridian that is being treated.

Sedation

Using a light touch, either with the fingertips or the whole hand, the meridian is massaged in the opposite direction to the energy flow, i.e. from the end point towards the Tsing point. The result is that excess energy is removed from the area or from the underlying cause. It is extremely influential where there is acute pain, spasm, heat and inflammation in the area, e.g. light touch massage along the course of the spleen meridian will help in all cases of uterine conditions. Several strokes along the meridian can be carried out and is most useful to perform at the commencement of a treatment.

Magnetism of the fingers

It has been mentioned several times, in different types of acupressure, that the practitioner places the *middle* finger of one hand on a point and the *middle* finger of the other hand on another point and then proceeds to balance the energy flow between them. Is it important to use these two fingers, and what is the significance in choosing them? 'Touch' therapists have argued in the past about which fingers are used in their particular discipline, and have given several reasons for the relative values of using the correct fingers.

It is said that each finger possesses either a negative or positive magnetic charge (see Figure 1.6). The charge of the thumbs is said to be neutral and they therefore have little influence in subtle energy balancing, although great significance in practical acupressure. The flow of electricity and magnetism is said to go from the negative pole towards the positive pole. This certainly appears to be the case in the human body. It appears that one side of the body has a negative magnetic charge and the other side has a

Figure 1.6 Magnetism of the hand.

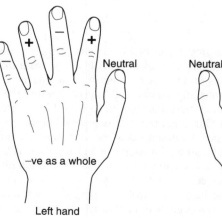
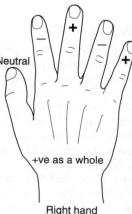

Left hand

Right hand

positive one. One whole hand is negatively charged and the other is positive. So it follows that, in order to create a balance of energy between two points, it is better for the therapist to hold with two fingers that have an opposite charge in order that energy may flow more easily. If it is impossible to use the same fingers, the balancing and hence treatment will still proceed, but at a slower rate.

Finally, a mention about cleanliness and hygiene. With all the techniques of acupressure that are used, personal cleanliness and hygiene has to be exemplary. Fingernails *must* be trimmed short. Also, with the whole range of different techniques that the therapist will perform, the hands have to be very soft as well as possibly being strong – so no rough skin. Please wear gloves when gardening and doing dirty work; always protect the hands and remember they are your livelihood.

2

The naturopathic assessment of disease

Before discussing how acupressure can be used to balance the body's energies, it is first necessary to discuss the important topics of naturopathic assessment of disease and what disease really is. Knowledge of naturopathy (of which acupressure is a part) is vital so that the practitioner can be fully equipped with the various energy changes taking place within the patient and how that can be utilized in a therapeutic way.

What is disease?

Many books have been written on this one topic alone, so below is a brief but salient explanation about disease. Disease should really be written down as dis-ease, as it represents a disharmony or 'ill at ease' in the body by whatever cause. Another way of describing dis-ease would be 'imbalance'. Therefore if the body is in a state of imbalance when it is sick, the purpose of acupressure (and other methods of healing) is to create balance from imbalance, or in other words to bring about a restoration of order or homoeostasis. The body is always attempting to show any trained person where the imbalance lies by producing symptoms of the disease and by creating signs that can be seen or palpated. It has to be stated loudly here that symptoms are *not* the disease itself but are external expressions and signs by the patient attempting to show a state of imbalance. Hippocrates stated quite categorically that symptoms are to be used 'like golden pearls' in order to reach a definitive diagnosis or analysis; symptoms should never be suppressed. Already it should be obvious to the reader that the naturopathic assessment of disease differs to that of conventional or orthodox (allopathic) medicine.

Disease is therefore considered to be an imbalance of vital force within and without the human frame. This is a fundamental precept, all else is meaningless, with it the nature of disease becomes clear. If any kind of unnatural, perverse or altered states of energy are introduced into the body, dis-ease will ensue. Philosophers down the ages have given this vital force different names and meanings and have attempted to quantify it. Hippocrates called it 'medicatrix naturae', Paracelsus called it 'archaeus', Mesmer called it 'animal magnetism', Von Reichenberg called it 'odic force', Palmer called it 'innate'. Traditional Eastern therapies know it as Prana, Ki or Chi.

There is a 'great divide' in considering disease aetiology, namely disease can either be inherited or acquired.

Inherited

It is common knowledge that humans are born with certain characteristics of their parents and grandparents, and that if, say, there was a history of asthma in the family, then the likelihood of the offspring falling to asthma would be more than if there was no heritable link. Scientists are slowly breaking down the complexities of the human genome, and eventually it will be possible to know what each and every gene is concerned with. Dr Charles Samuel Hahnemann had never heard of genes. He was a German medical scientist (1755–1843) and had a reputation of being one of the most brilliant chemists and physicians in Germany at that time. As his experience grew, he became more and more dissatisfied with the current medical practice which consisted largely of bleeding and purging the patient or forcing him to swallow large draughts of drug mixtures. After a few years experiencing these methods, Hahnemann felt that the cure of the disease or even the restoration of health was so problematic that he was compelled to give up his medical practice and began to earn his living by translating works on chemistry and medicine. In 1790 he was translating an English *Materia Medica* into German and found that he could not agree with the explanation of the action of cinchona bark in the cure of malaria. He took the very brave step of taking the poison cinchona himself. He wanted to know what reaction this drug would have on a person who was well. He suffered some bad symptoms over the next 4 hours, weariness in the limbs, trembling, head pounding, redness, sweating and thirst – in other words all the classical symptoms of malaria. He could not rationalize how taking the tincture of cinchona could *give* symptoms similar to malaria in a well person whilst at the same time the books said that it cured the disease! He then, with colleagues, took various substances, belladonna, poison ivy, various salts etc. and made a note of the findings. In each case the symptoms of the disease occurred when the drug was taken and they became well when they stopped taking it. They had discovered the naturopathic law of similars – *similia curenter similibus* – which translated from the Latin means 'let likes be cured by likes'. What he proceeded to do then is nothing short of divine inspiration at the most, and astonishing at the very least. He studied the writings of Hippocrates and Paracelsus on the subject of the *dynamism* or *vital force* in a substance. So he tried to extricate the dynamism or vital force from the remedy. He took 1 ml of the original tincture and placed it in 9 ml of water, shook it, put it into a centrifuge and succussed it. The resultant mixture he called the first potency. He repeated this procedure until the resultant 'medicine' became more and more dilute, and yet seemingly more and more powerful. In our present homoeopathic remedies, the lowest potency that one would normally use in therapy would be 6x potency (the procedure repeated six times). If dilution, succussion, centrifugation and shaking continues to be carried out, something 'magical' occurs at 11.5 c potency (a 'c' potency is when 1 ml of the original substance is diluted in 99 ml of water or spirit). All trace of the original substance disappears, and yet in continued dilution the potency becomes more powerful. This point is called 'Avogadro's point'. When it is considered that commonly used remedies are 30 c, 100 c (1 M), 10 M etc. then it can quickly be seen that this is entering the realms of *energy medicine*. In order to understand both the cause and cure of disease, it is essential to understand that it is the vital force of the human body that is changed by remedies to effect changes of symptoms and hence changes of illness and constitutions. 'Subtle is powerful': this phrase is just as apt in acupressure as it is in homoeopathy.

Hahnemann's work then took him into trying to ascertain the cause of disease and he spent over 40 years of his life in that quest. He stated that dis-ease is mostly inherited by what he called miasms or taints of dis-ease. In other words, he believed that we are all born with a predisposition to some kind of dis-ease factor depending on our hereditary background. His work concluded that there are three major miasms – psora, syphilis and sycosis. He said that psora represented the original dis-ease pattern in the human race (some scholars have deduced this as meaning 'original sin'), this governs some skin problems and respiratory conditions. In the early to mid centuries, the venereal diseases of syphilis and gonorrhoea raised their ugly heads and in turn were treated by suppressive means, thus driving the disease force deeper into the constitution of man and becoming part of the miasmitic chain, the taint or predisposition of which are passed on from generation to generation. The syphilitic miasm gives conditions associated with bony deformities, indurations and ulcerations with nightly aggravations. The sycotic (gonorrhoeal) gives rise to conditions affecting the nervous system, also some skin problems, warts and mental imbalance. The combined miasms then appeared after a few generations of suppression of dis-ease. Psora combined with syphilis is called the tubercular miasm and gives us the classical tubercular constitution of respiratory and bone conditions, lethargy and some mental conditions. This group of people are usually allergic to bovine foods, i.e. milk, cheese etc. and are prone to catarrh. The psora–sycosis combination is called the arthritis miasm and governs those people who have inherited the rheumatoid factor. When all three miasms are active, the disease process is most chronic, giving a greater deterioration of vital force, e.g. the cancers, HIV and other chronic disease. So, in summary, according to Hahnemann and the laws of constitutional homoeopathy, we all have a predisposition to disease. A person can go through his or her life without any symptoms whatsoever, but if the vital force is rattled, as in shock (mental or physical), grief, a virus or prolonged stress as in emotional stress or eating the wrong foods over a period of time, then the predisposition or the miasm becomes symptomatic. Hahnemann used a wonderful phrase to describe this – 'the miasm is raised'. Further miasms have been introduced into the races in the twentieth century by the constant and repetitive suppression of vital force. These have probably come about because of mass inoculation and vaccination, the use of antibiotics and the birth pill.

The story of Hahnemann and the theory of inherited disease according to him and subsequent classical homoeopathic philosophy has been purposely laboured and may seem, to some, to be a strange inclusion in a textbook on acupressure. It was included for two reasons.

First, to introduce the more orthodox therapist to the important theories of inherited disease and how they affect our thinking when it comes to planning a treatment regime, for instance when the therapist is confronted with chronic dis-ease, it is essential to appreciate that there is a limitation of recovery expectation because of the predisposed weakness. In acupressure terms, the Yin organ/meridians of kidney, spleen, lung and liver (but especially kidney) must be stimulated prior to treatment of any chronic condition – this will be covered in detail in Chapter 4.

Secondly, to try and show the reader that clinical acupressure, when performed as a total treatment regimen comes under the umbrella of naturopathic and holistic medicine, which is a far cry from the various methods taught on many weekend courses and told in several paperback books on the subject. Acupressure should not be perceived as just the 'twiddling' of a particular acupoint in order to create pain relief at a distant area. It is a much more noble art form than that.

Acquired

The list of dis-ease that is acquired is probably endless. In each and every case of acquired dis-ease there is an imbalance of the vital force within and without the body by external means which causes internal chaos. There is a term used in some 'New Age' circles that *all is energy*. This means that everything about the Earth and all its inhabitants (including human beings) can be described in various energy (vital force) terms of frequency, wavelength, colour, sound, thought and touch, and that anything the human body is subjected to of an alien or obnoxious nature can result in an energy imbalance which will eventually produce dis-ease. Below are some acquired causes of dis-ease and medical conditions.

1. Hygiene

Good hygiene is a prerequisite for good health and energetic harmony. Failure to keep to good hygienic practices can lead to all manner of germ-related disease including cholera, dysentery etc. Although it is unlikely that the practitioner would have to deal with such imbalance when using acupressure, it is essential that a complete and thorough case sheet is taken so that a history of such disease can be omitted. If there is a history of bad hygiene in the family, the lung meridian is stimulated to boost the excretory system and the spleen meridian is stimulated in order to boost the immune system.

2. Viruses

When dealing with dis-ease of a viral aetiology, it is essential that the lung, spleen and large intestine meridians are stimulated in order to assist the body's excretory and immune systems. This is particularly apt after the patient has been through a prolonged bout of influenza or respiratory virus. If left unattended, these can play havoc with the system and can lead to very unpleasant symptoms, most of which can be avoided by good 'hands-on' therapy.

3. Chemical ingestion

Much research has been carried out recently into the effects of too much ingestion of various chemicals or the giving of vaccinations that seem to cause unpleasant side effects. Reference is made particularly to 'Gulf war syndrome' and the ingestion of organophosphates. Why these chemicals can cause so much chaos in the system has been a mystery to allopathic medicine, but can be answered very well by traditional Chinese medicine (TCM). This will be covered later on in this chapter when dis-ease as a 'force' will be discussed and how this force affects various internal organs. In acupressure treatment terms, again, it is the lung and spleen meridians that need to be boosted initially followed by treatment of the individual organ that has been affected.

4. Iatrogenic (synthetic and chemical drugs)

This is where the patient has been subjected to too many chemical and synthetic drugs given in all good faith by their physicians. What was once considered to be an irrelevance is now thought to be a major cause of imbalance. There are many differences of attitude and philosophy between naturopathic and allopathic medicine. Two differences that spring to mind when attempting to explain why some patients are so badly affected by the prolonged taking of some drugs are (a) Modern medicine tends to compartmentalize the body into various systems and organs without the vision that health and harmony is dependent upon a good energy balance occurring with all the organs. The giving of specifically acting drugs to affect individual organs over a long period of time is bound to have knock on effects with other organs, there is no option. (b) Allopathic medicines almost always treat the symptoms of the disease and not necessarily the dis-ease process itself. This has adverse affects in that the cause of the disharmony is not addressed and that synthetic drugs tend to have a suppressing effect on the vital force of the person. Thankfully the human body is always attempting to heal itself with its own built-in energy system and can cope with very many drugs and other toxins that are thrown at it, but there comes a time when disease force starts to win – that is what happens in iatrogenic disease. When using acupressure, it is vital that the liver and spleen energies are built up before addressing any specific symptom.

5. Accidents and injuries

This particular cause of dis-ease and medical conditions was mentioned in the last book, but it would be of benefit here to discuss this topic in a different way. In the book *Acupressure: Clinical Applications in Musculo-skeletal Conditions* it was stated that there are many seemingly mechanical conditions that could be caused by a combination of pathological, hormonal and emotional factors. This time, a few examples will be given of how mechanical imbalances in the body can give rise to pathological conditions.

Figure 2.1 shows the 'healing triad'. In naturopathic medicine, the human body is considered to be made up of equal measures of mechanical, mental and chemical parts, each dependent on the others for support and energy. If one system starts to fail, it *will* affect the other two. The severity of the effect depends mostly upon the constitutional health of the person. Examples of how some mechanical conditions can be the cause of medical conditions are as follows. (a) A lesion around the shoulder that is either not treated correctly or not treated at all could become a 'frozen' shoulder. This

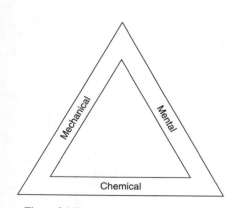

Figure 2.1 The healing triad.

in turn affects the flow of energy, nerve conduction, blood circulation and lymph that passes through and around the shoulder, which in turn can produce acute dis-ease changes in the large intestine (constipation), lungs (tightness in the chest) and gall bladder. These three meridians pass close to the shoulder and are affected to some degree or another and will eventually cause conditions in their corresponding organs. (b) A chronic untreated lesion of the ankle joint, especially where there has been a traumatic inversion sprain can eventually give problems with the bladder. In applied kinesiology, the peroneus longus muscle (the muscle that everts the ankle) is associated with the bladder meridian, similarly the end of the bladder meridian is situated over the lateral aspect of the foot and is badly affected in ankle sprains. There tends to be a sluggishness that builds up within the bladder system that can cause weakness of the spine as a whole, also sluggishness of urine flow and prostatitis. (c) Any lesion of the spine may give rise to blood, lymphatic, nerve and energy flow as well as joint changes. Traditional Chinese medicine states that most vertebrae are associated with the energy to specific organs (associated effect points). It is thought that these are linked via the autonomic nervous system. Some of the AEPs will be mentioned later in the chapter when naturopathic assessment is discussed. The AEPs also form part of the modern way of looking at the association of the physical body and the emotions.

The art of analysis by psychoimmunotherapy or 'mind–body' therapy has become more accepted over the past 5 years by the establishment as being a valid diagnostic tool. This concept will be mentioned several times later in this book and, hopefully, will be the subject of a book of mine in due course.

6. Drugs

It is a well known fact that the ongoing use of leisure drugs such as alcohol, tobacco and cannabis, for example, can greatly affect the vital force of a person. Whether or not they cause chronic dis-ease, e.g. lung or liver cancer is totally dependent upon the person's constitution and general predispositional weakness or strength. In acupressure, it is important that we know if our patient is a smoker or heavy drinker as their disease process could have caused their particular symptoms. The lung meridian should be stimulated in the case of smoking and the liver meridian in the case of drinking.

7. Air pollution

The effects of air and other forms of pollution have become more widespread over the past few years. The burning of fossil fuels and their discharge of toxins into the atmosphere has given rise to some serious dis-ease patterns in humans and animals. It is a fact that there is far more asthma and other respiratory illnesses now than there has ever been. More and more people are striving for cleaner air and are trying to leave the big cities for country or seaside life where there seems to be more fresh air. In acupressure, if our patients are affected by pollution, the lung meridian should be heavily stimulated so as to aid the elimination of respiratory toxins, plus the spleen and stomach meridians so as to boost the immune system and general energy of the patient.

8. Food and drink

This is another topic that complete books have been written about. There is a hackneyed expression that 'you are what you eat'. This phrase was introduced in the early 1970s and was greeted with typical apathy by the medical establishment. The idea that the food we ate could have any bearing on our health was scorned. I well remember in the mid-1970s, whilst working in the NHS, the scores of children I treated who had various forms of juvenile arthritis. As well as my physiotherapy treatments of providing joint mobilizing, wax baths, infrared, splints and walking re-education, I attempted to perform some acupressure and reflexology techniques on these poorly mites. They seemed to respond very well to this, but to my horror, at most meal times they were served up lashings of sausages and other red meats plus lots of cream and sugary foods (as a treat!). I often wonder how much more damage was done to them as their systems attempted to cope with all the extra acid-forming foods. It was bad enough for them to have to cope with their mega doses of steroids and gold injections!

I do not expect any therapist reading this book to be versed in all aspects of naturopathic nutrition, but it would be beneficial for them to study this subject. There has been an explosion of information over the past 20 years with regard to the food that we eat being responsible for health patterns. My personal feeling is that there is too much information available, much of which is contradictory. The consumer does not know where they stand any more. The following represents the salient points of what every health-care professional should be aware of whilst treating their patients. They should be able to disseminate this common knowledge to their patients in order to augment their treatment: (a) cut out white sugar and red meat in cases of arthritis and people who have the rheumatoid factor, (b) cut out white flour products and yeast in people who have bowel disease, (c) cut out dairy produce to all those who have catarrh, sinus trouble or respiratory problems. It is also a simple maxim that in most cases of ill health, in order for the body to restore health, self-healing is engendered by eating whole foods and by cutting out preservatives and additives. In acupressure, to aid the patient's digestive energy, the stomach, small intestine, large intestine and spleen meridians should be stimulated either prior to treatment or sometimes during it.

9. Adverse radiation

This can be a controversial topic and its airing in public can bring about much derision. There is no doubt in my mind though that adverse radiation in all its forms can and does affect the vital force, hence giving symptoms and dis-ease patterns. It will not necessarily affect the acupressure treatment, but it is advisable for the therapist to be aware that adverse radiation aetiology could be the aspect of disharmony that may have been overlooked in the assessment. It has already been stated that the human frame is energy – therefore if it is subjected to adverse or 'bad' energy, it is bound to be affected and to become sick.

It is staggering in the extreme how medical science still persists in denying the facts. It surely cannot be a coincidence that there are concentrated cases of cancer and birth defects in people who live close to overhead power cables and nuclear power stations. Adverse radiation doesn't just cause serious illness though – my experience has shown that some people can be badly affected with catarrh, sinusitis, migraine, headaches and general lethargy by using computers and other types of VDU, or by sitting for too long in front of televisions, using microwaves and photocopy machines. The perverse radiations do not affect everyone, just those who are prone and have a predisposed sensitivity or allergy. Particular adverse radiation affects specific parts of the body as they are 'ingested' into the physical body via the chakras. It is the throat chakra (Vishudda) that is affected mostly, thus giving symptoms that affect the body's excretory and eliminative systems. This is a huge topic and one that will be covered in my book on 'Healing with the Chakra Energy System'. In acupressure, if adverse radiation seems to be the cause of the patient's ill health, the large intestine and lung meridians should be stimulated prior to treatment.

10. Shock

It has already been stated that we all have predispositional patterns of health. Depending upon the constitution and lifestyle of the person, the taints of dis-ease could be latent for a lifetime and do not become symptomatic. It takes, however, some kind of jolt or shudder to the system in order to 'raise the miasm' or for the taint to become active and to start to affect the physical body. Shock, either physical or emotional, has a powerful effect on the human frame. The therapist must see scores of cases in a single year when the patient will say 'I have not been well since…'. The 'since' is the turning point or watershed in their lives when the shock to the system first took place. When practising as a homoeopath, I used to give a dose of high potency arnica to attempt to antidote the shock. It occasionally needed a different remedy. The Bach flower composite 'Rescue Remedy' is sometimes needed. There is, however, no orthodox medical treatment for shock that is as rapid and effective as homoeopathic arnica.

11. Ultraviolet

This topic would probably not have been included a few years ago. Since we have become aware of global warming and the burning of fossil fuels causing 'holes' in the ozone layer, it is now apparent that people can be badly affected by too much ultraviolet on the skin. There have always been the dangers of burning the skin, but now there are very real dangers that conditions such as skin cancer can be caused by ultraviolet exposure. The use of acupressure in such diseases is not as effective as allopathic treatments with the exception of using stimulating massage on the spleen, lung and kidney meridians in order to boost the immune and excretory systems.

12. Cold and heat

This represents a major source of energy imbalance in the body. If the reader would care to read *Su Wen Nei Ching* or *The Yellow Emperor's Classic of Internal Medicine* (translated by Ilza Veith), it will soon become clear that according to TCM, the vast majority of dis-ease is caused by external weather influences. Examples of these are: cold which affects the flow of energy to the kidneys, heat which affects the heart and small intestine, and damp which affects the spleen. Even the direction of the wind is an important factor as to which organ is influenced. The law of five elements or transformations (which is one of the amazing natural laws of naturopathic and traditional medicine) fully explains these phenomena. It is therefore very important to get a full case history from the patient to include any episodes of them being affected by the weather. It is equally important to use the correct acupressure treatment to try and compensate for it and to strengthen the body's reserves. These will be explained later.

13. Negative thought

Earlier on, the phrase 'You are what you eat' was used to explain that the food we eat has a vital influence on our disease processes. An equally important phrase is 'You become what you think'. It is now accepted that much physical dis-ease can be caused by continued negative emotions. 'Thought' is a powerful tool when used as a positive and negative force. Thought, like everything else to do with the human body, can be considered as manifestations of Chi energy, and as such can influence the person's energy body. Generally speaking, we feel better when we engender positive thoughts and we feel worse when we are negative. It is the constant negative emotional thoughts of depression, anxiety, grief, sadness, guilt etc. that affect our physical bodies. This is such an important subject that this book has included a whole chapter on the cause and treatment of stress and stress-related conditions, and its treatment using acupressure.

Naturopathic assessment

Before treatment can commence, it is vital to ascertain a treatment regimen dependent upon the presented symptoms. As stated before, it is imperative for the therapist to take a good, salient case history – do not allow the patient to 'waffle', make sure they stick strictly to the exact history. Taking a good case history is an art form in its own right. Following the case history will be the physical examination. Even though the therapist will have a good idea as to what systems, meridians and organs are affected, it is essential to undergo a complete naturopathic assessment as there are sometimes a few surprises that come to the fore that were not apparent in the question and answer session. When it comes to physical examination, it must be carried out in comfortable, warm surroundings. Nothing is worse for the patient than to be lying on the couch with next to nothing on and to be freezing cold! The assessment can be roughly divided into two sections. The first is to do with *looking*, the second deals with *feeling*. The following represent the areas of the body that need to looked at and felt before a definitive diagnosis and final analysis can be made:

Looking – (a) tongue and (b) face.
Feeling – (a) pulse, (b) abdomen, (c) foot reflexes, (d) hand reflexes, (e) meridian end points and (f) listening posts.

A more complete analysis would probably include iris diagnosis and auriculotherapy, but both of these represent months, if not years, of study to perfect. The eight areas of analysis chosen are sufficient for the practitioner of acupressure. If the reader is interested in iris diagnosis and auriculotherapy, they have been included in my chapter on naturopathic assessment in the book *Complementary Therapies for Physical Therapists* (2000). For those practitioners who have made an in-depth study of these two types of diagnosis, they can still be used to great effect as back-up analysis and confirmation of previous findings.

The eight areas of 'look' and 'feel' can be likened to a microcosm within the macrocosm. Each of the areas is said to be reflected areas of the whole and as such represent the whole of the body in miniature. Reflected areas show where the body's energy imbalance lies – it is as if the patient were attempting to wave a flag in an effort to communicate knowledge to the practitioner. It never ceases to amaze me how the body is capable of doing this. It is a very accurate system of diagnosis and analysis and relatively simple to learn. It is such a pity that allopathically trained medical personnel choose to ignore or denigrate it.

Looking

(a) Tongue

Tongue diagnosis is one of the cornerstones of traditional Chinese and Japanese medicine and has therefore been with us for at least 5000 years. It is said that the tongue in general terms is the outward expression of the stomach. This means that any imbalance within the digestive system can easily be detected in the tongue. The tongue will remain furred with white or yellow coating so long as the stomach remains in a state of imbalance. When we fast, as the body attempts to get rid of accumulated toxins and poisons, the tongue will slowly change from having a very white and 'yucky' appearance to that of being nice and pink. Traditionally, we are supposed to fast for as long as the tongue remains furred – not many of us are that brave though! Much more though than representing the stomach and digestion (as it is used in modern medicine), the tongue also represents the many areas of the body, similarly to the other reflected areas. It is a most reliable indicator and changes to it often occur within a few hours of changes in the physical body. By observing the tongue, the therapist can observe the dis-ease progression and therefore it is useful to observe the patient's tongue at each and every visit. Observation of the tongue consists of two parts, the body of the tongue and the coating. The body of the tongue is a useful guide in chronic dis-ease and the coating is used to analyse acute conditions.

Body of tongue – A pale white tongue represents an empty cold condition with insufficient Yang energy to push the blood up. A scarlet or red body indicates heat in the person – the more red it is, the hotter the condition. A purple tongue is a serious condition that involves stagnant blood due to weak Chi.

Coating – A white coating indicates excess water internally; if greasy it indicates damp heat with problems with the stomach or spleen. A yellow coating indicates a worsening of the disease process or an infection in the part represented by the area of yellowing. A black or grey coating is a more serious disease. This involves kidney Chi and is said to be a cold disease.

Figure 2.2 Tongue diagnosis.

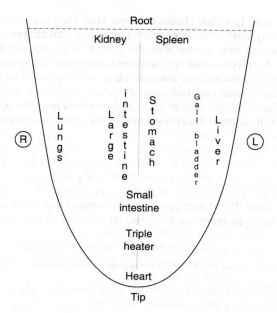

Tongue areas

Figure 2.2 shows a diagram of the areas of the tongue. As with most of the other reflected areas of the body, the middle of the tongue is associated with the 'middle' of the person, i.e. the stomach and bowel. The tip of the tongue represents the 'Fire' organs of the heart, triple heater and small intestine and the root of the tongue represents the deep organs of the kidney and spleen. The right side represents the lungs and the left side the liver. Red patches that appear on these various areas indicate that there is an inflammatory process taking place in the particular organ. This could be due to an infection, healing crisis or aggravation or generalized Yang condition. The meridian associated with the organ in question needs to be sedated. If the body of the tongue is dull, white and slippery, the underlying Yin condition will need to be addressed by stimulating the associated meridian. This technique will be discussed in a future chapter.

(b) Face

Facial diagnosis represents another facet of traditional diagnosis that has been used for centuries. There is much information to be gleaned from carefully examining the face. Figure 2.3 shows a diagram of the face and the associated organic areas.

Facial colour

A chalky white complexion means a general deficiency of Chi and coldness with a possible condition of the respiratory system. A generalized

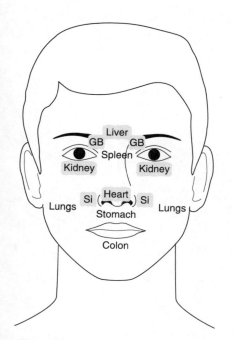

Figure 2.3 Facial diagnosis.

red colour (not just the cheeks) means that there is much Yang or heat in the system – it may also indicate a circulatory imbalance. A yellow appearance means that there is a deficiency of Chi in the stomach and spleen, with or without dampness. A greenish tinge indicates liver disharmony, internal cold or pain. A blackish tinge, especially under the eyes, indicates a 'water' imbalance and a possible kidney condition. Please note that the different colours associated with the imbalances follow the colours used in the law of the five transformations or elements.

Facial diagnostic areas

There are several different interpretations of this. They differ according to the traditional philosophy, i.e. Chinese, Japanese or Ayurvedic.

Lungs: Located on the cheeks. A white discoloration indicates Chi deficiency, whereas a reddish colour represents heat or inflammation. The more chronic the respiratory condition, e.g. emphysema, the whiter will be the colour.

Bronchi: Situated on the nostrils: white nostrils indicate a chronic complaint, whereas redness indicates heat and inflammation.

Large intestine: This organ is represented on the lower lip and the jaw. Swelling of the lower lip may indicate weakness of Chi in the large bowel and its incapability of ridding the body of toxins. Dryness indicates a lack of fluid in the bowel. Red indicates heat and inflammation. Most problems with the large bowel that are indicated in the face can usually be cleared with the correct dietary advice.

Stomach: This is located midway along the bridge of the nose and on the upper lip. Swelling of the upper lip indicates disharmony in the stomach, in that there is probably toxins that the stomach is attempting to deal with, or that there may be an imbalance in the protein–fat relationship. Dryness and cracking indicates stomach Chi deficiency. Yellowing indicates a general weakness in the digestive system, with particular emphasis on the possibility of allergies and candidiasis.

Spleen: This is located on the bridge of the nose up towards the eyes. Yellowing in that area almost certainly indicates allergies and a weakness in the immune system. Serrated lines along the bridge of the nose indicates a long term (chronic) imbalance and could indicate a severe immune disease. A darkish colour would indicate weak spleen Chi.

Liver: This is located between the eyebrows around the 'third eye' point. Furrows and lines there may indicate a chronic organic imbalance and/or allergy of the non-food variety, e.g. hay fever. A redness indicates inflammation of the more acute type.

Gall bladder: Located on the eyelids. Redness here indicates a Yang condition, e.g. cholecystitis. The writer has occasionally been able to tell the patient of the possibility of calculi in the gall bladder, as there appears tiny hard nodules on the eyelids, not to be confused with either styes or localized lymphatic obstructions.

Nervous system: This is represented as a large area on the forehead. Many vertical lines in this area could indicate a weakness in the nervous system such as worry and stress-related problems. The patient's age, obviously, has to be taken into account. As with every other area of diagnosis, facial analysis should *not* be taken out of context but used as just part of the *whole* picture.

Figure 2.4 Pulse diagnosis.

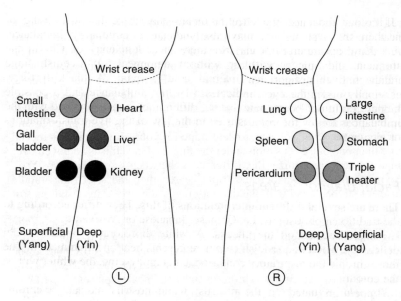

Feeling

(a) Pulse

The pulse diagnosis (Figure 2.4) represents one of the oldest types of traditional diagnosis. It can be very complicated to learn in detail, but can be mastered if learnt slowly over the weeks and months. It is not something that is assimilated easily and the practitioner must practice constantly to achieve the desired results. Physiotherapists and other orthodox practitioners are used to the knowledge of having just *one* pulse at the distal end of the radial artery by the wrist. To be told that there are 12 interpretations of this one pulse can go against one's basic beliefs, and when one commences to try and find the pulse differences, one is all 'thumbs'. Slowly but surely, however, these subtle differences can be felt. Reading the pulse according to traditional Chinese and Japanese medicine can provide much needed information about the patient's entire constitutional condition. So-called acupuncturists and acupressure therapists who are only wedded to Western beliefs and who mainly perform symptomatic 'pin pricking' and pressure techniques do not know what they are missing without this extra knowledge.

To take the pulse, ensure the patient's arm is horizontal and the wrist is lower than the heart. The therapist should use three fingers placed on the patient's pulse just above the wrist crease. The left hand pulse is usually stronger in men and the right hand pulse is stronger in women. The fingers should, one by one, be pressed down to almost occlude the flow of blood and then released slightly – this gives the deeper or the Yin pulse. The superficial or Yang pulse is felt by a gentle touch of the finger on the radial artery. At each of the six sites there is a Yin and Yang association which is coupled with the energetic quality of the corresponding internal organ.

If it is just about acceptable for the sceptical orthodox therapist to accept that there are 12 pulses, not *one*, it really stretches credulity to the limit to think that there are up to 27 variations of each of the 12. The pulse can be superficial, floating, deep, slow, rapid, empty, full, slippery, choppy, thready, fine, thin, tight, wiry, weak, etc. Each one of these different variations is significant in the overall picture of the patient's condition. They are far too elaborate and complicated to discuss here. The easy way for the practitioner to appreciate the different pulses is to practice and practice on whoever you can, to determine for yourself that there is indeed more than one pulse sensation under the fingers. Once this is achieved over time, try and recognize the differences between, say, the two Yang proximal pulses of bladder and triple heater, then the two Yang middle pulses of stomach and gall bladder and finally the two Yang distal ones of large intestine and small intestine. Repeat this with the Yin pulses. Do not at first try and feel a difference between a Yin pulse and its corresponding Yang one. Try and feel the differences between like and like first of all. Only then will you be able to start to feel the many subtle differences. The overriding sensations that the therapist must feel in analysis is the difference between empty (chronic) and full (acute) pulses. When this difference is mastered, it will give a tremendous boost to the analytical skills and the ability to be able to treat the patient correctly, not just by palliating the symptoms.

(b) Abdomen

The study and practice of abdominal diagnosis can be divided into two types – the hara diagnosis and the alarm points.

Hara diagnosis

The abdomen is divided into reflected areas or reflexes that correspond with the associated organs. There exists several different charts and interpretations of Hara diagnosis and the one in Figure 2.5 shows a composite view. It is the one that the author has used and taught for several years. If the therapist presses the associated area with a gentle touch and elicits pain or discomfort in the area, this usually indicates an acute inflammatory state in the associated organ. Steps must be taken to address this situation as the initial part of the treatment. It is usual to sedate the source point of the organ concerned. This should alleviate the acute symptoms (this technique is shown in Chapter 4). Pain and discomfort found with a much deeper palpation indicates a more chronic and long-standing condition and organic imbalance. In this instance, the information is used as part of the whole picture and a treatment regimen is calculated using this information together with all the other collated information.

There is often some obvious changes to the abdominal areas that show readily that there is some kind of imbalance, namely, tension of the tissues, heat and redness, inflammation on and under the skin, and swelling of the area. When the patient shows an absolute hatred of the abdomen being touched at all, this often indicates a deep-seated emotional imbalance. Abdominal diagnosis areas are always referred to, in the various texts, as being only of analytical value. The author has, though, for several years

Figure 2.5 Abdominal diagnosis.

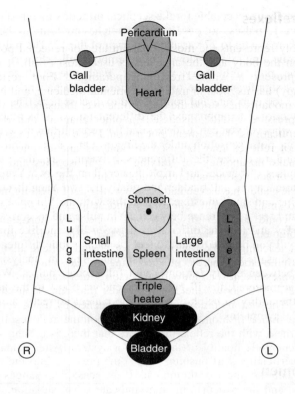

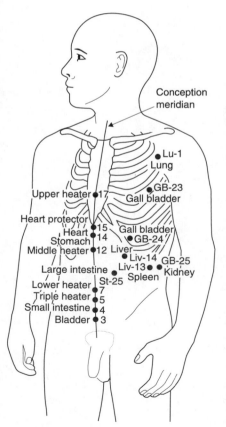

Figure 2.6 Abdominal alarm points.

practised and taught the Hara points as a mode of treatment. This can be achieved by using two techniques, either energy balance the area with another reflex associated with the same organ or balance it with the source point of the associated meridian. Where the reflected area is a large one, the whole of the hand may be placed over it. This method is shown in Chapter 4.

Alarm points

The alarm points (Figure 2.6) are often called the front collecting points or mo points. They represent acutely painful 'trigger' spots when the associated organ is in a state of acute imbalance. Like the hara points, these points can also be used in treatment mode as well as in analysis. If the point is very acute, it can be energy balanced with another reflected point of the organ (foot, hand, scalp, hara, ear etc.) or with the source point of the meridian. If the point is not too tender, it is also possible to gently massage it with a gentle but firm constant pressure using a short rotational massage technique. This can be an extremely effective way of balancing the energy in the organ.

The hara and alarm points are excellent energy indicators as well as being useful treatment tools. As with all reflected points and pathways (reflexes) they represent the microcosm of the macrocosm. What is the patient attempting to tell us? How can we best find out what is the root cause of their condition?

(c) Foot reflexes

This probably represents the most important area of reflected points and pathways on the body and the area that is used most of all. It does, of course, represent a whole treatment paradigm. Foot reflexology (reflextherapy) has its roots in traditional oriental medicine, and its use as a treatment modality has stood the test of time over thousands of years. Its use in acupressure will be discussed in other chapters that deal with practical applications of treatment, but it would be useful here to mention how the foot reflexes may be used in analysis and diagnosis. Firstly though, I make no apology for 'mixing' the philosophies and practical applications of acupressure and reflexology. This would seen to be heresy in some circles, and I have even had people walk out of a lecture indicating to me in no small way that reflexology and acupressure should remain separate. I would consider this viewpoint to be very short-sighted and somewhat bigoted. I have been using these two philosophies together in clinical and teaching work for over 25 years and believe that each is stronger with the other. There is no such thing as 'classical' reflexology or classical acupressure, just an individual person's interpretation of each art!

Figures 2.7–2.10 shows the main reflexes that can be used by the practitioner. The various reflexes should be touched by using very gentle pressure in a similar fashion to palpating the abdominal reflexes. If there is acute tenderness with the reflex, this shows that there is a Yang situation within the energetic quality of the organ or system. After palpating the reflexes superficially, start pushing with some pressure into the reflected area either with the finger or thumb pad. If the sensation changes (both to the therapist and the patient), this may indicate a Yin situation. The Yin reflex sensation has a far duller and more diffuse feeling to that of the Yang sensation, and the difference is only appreciated with experience. It is best to palpate all the organs superficially and to await response from the patient each time, before proceeding to the deeper palpation. The patient will become confused and could suffer from 'reflex palpation indigestion' if both superficial and deep palpation were done on the same organ. Try it sometime and see what I mean! Where the organ is represented by quite a large reflected area on the foot, e.g. lung, it will be necessary to choose just one point in the middle of the reflected area or the area where the patient is complaining of discomfort. With experience of doing this technique, it is best to work down the feet starting at the top and proceeding downwards but keeping to the same system of reflexes, also start on the right foot first. The order of the reflexes palpated therefore would be:

1. Great toe reflexes covering the brain and upper part of the central nervous system, followed by each vertebra in turn from the atlas to the coccyx (this is only possible if you are an experienced reflexologist).
2. Pituitary, hypothalamus, thyroid, parathyroid, thymus, solar plexus, adrenals.
3. Sinuses, eyes and ears.
4. Throat and oesophagus.
5. Lung, bronchus, diaphragm and heart.
6. Central organs of stomach, small intestine, pancreas, gall bladder and liver (spleen on the left foot).
7. Kidney, urethra, bladder and ureter.
8. Large bowel, ileo-caecal valve (ICV), sigmoid colon and rectum.

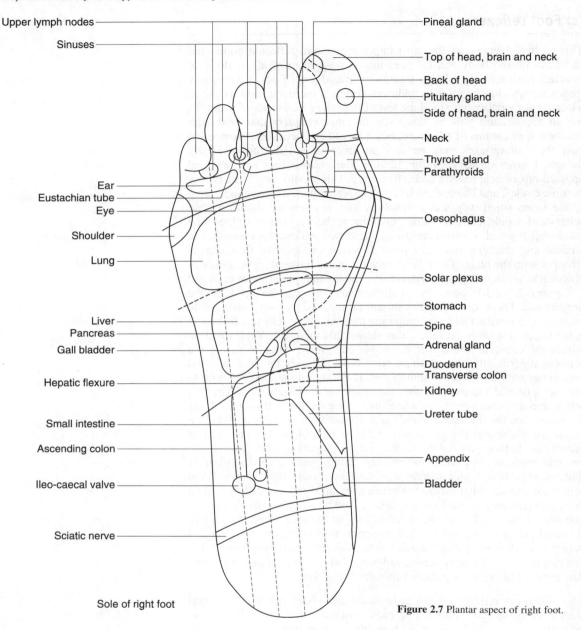

Upper lymph nodes
Sinuses

Pineal gland
Top of head, brain and neck
Back of head
Pituitary gland
Side of head, brain and neck
Neck
Thyroid gland
Parathyroids

Ear
Eustachian tube
Eye
Shoulder
Lung

Oesophagus

Solar plexus

Stomach
Liver
Pancreas
Spine
Gall bladder
Adrenal gland
Duodenum
Transverse colon
Hepatic flexure
Kidney

Small intestine
Ureter tube

Ascending colon
Ileo-caecal valve
Appendix
Bladder

Sciatic nerve

Sole of right foot

Figure 2.7 Plantar aspect of right foot.

9.   Pelvic region, sciatic nerve, testes and ovaries.
10. Lymphatic areas on the dorsum of the foot.

It is also possible to palpate the energetic quality in each of the joints and major muscle bulks with this technique.

After the above procedure, which should only take a couple of minutes, the analytical picture should be building up in your mind. The last two procedures of 'feel' should reinforce what the other reflexes have shown you; it would be unusual if something new were presented, but it does

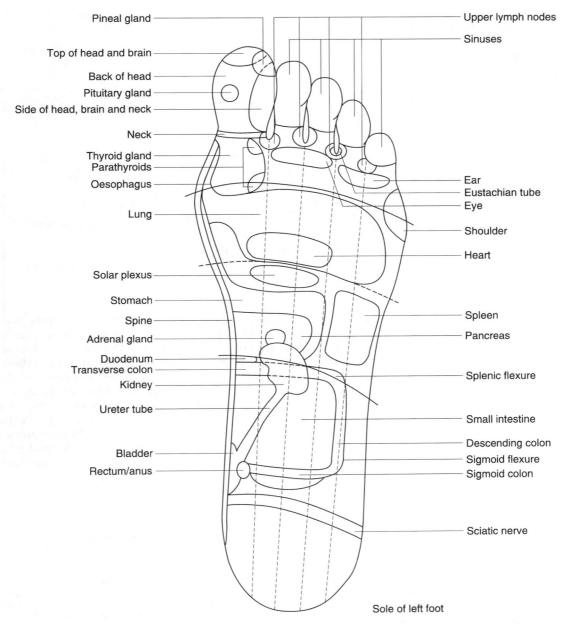

Pineal gland
Top of head and brain
Back of head
Pituitary gland
Side of head, brain and neck
Neck
Thyroid gland
Parathyroids
Oesophagus
Lung
Solar plexus
Stomach
Spine
Adrenal gland
Duodenum
Transverse colon
Kidney
Ureter tube
Bladder
Rectum/anus

Upper lymph nodes
Sinuses
Ear
Eustachian tube
Eye
Shoulder
Heart
Spleen
Pancreas
Splenic flexure
Small intestine
Descending colon
Sigmoid flexure
Sigmoid colon
Sciatic nerve

Sole of left foot

Figure 2.8 Plantar aspect of left foot.

happen occasionally, so it is best to carry out the remainder of the analysis at the end. Try not to cut corners.

(d) Hand reflexology

Hand reflexology is a much underrated art and has taken a back seat in popularity with its more popular cousin, foot reflexology. Recently, however, it has become much more popular and is being taught at most

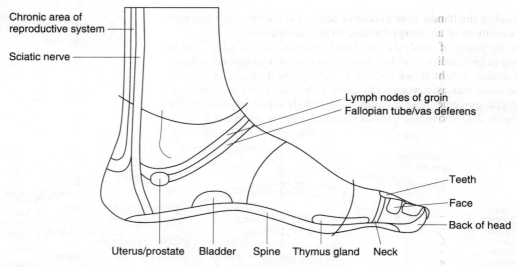

Figure 2.9 Medial aspect of left foot.

mainstream reflexology schools. In foot reflexology, points needing treatment are tender, and the reflexes on the hand will also be tender if the associated part of the body is in a state of imbalance and subsequently needs treatment. The reflexes on the hand, though, will not exhibit the same degree of acute tenderness as the ones on the feet because the hands are in everyday use much more than the feet and therefore reflexes become 'hidden'. The great beauty of hand reflexology is in the use of self-treatment. It is far easier to teach a patient how to massage specific points and areas on his or her hands than to massage the feet. In my opinion, it is not so important to introduce a holistic approach with the hand reflexes, therefore the patient can easily be taught how to gently massage the

Figure 2.10 Anterior-lateral aspect of left foot.

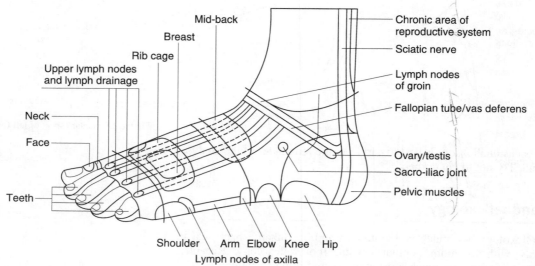

various areas of the hands, how to relieve acute and chronic pain and also how to create more of an energy balance to the injured area.

For the purposes of analysis, the hand reflexes are of more use in determining acute conditions rather than chronic ones. The various reflexes may be palpated in whichever order the therapist desires and is done in exactly the same way as palpating the foot reflexes in acute conditions, i.e. gentle circular movements in an attempt to initiate some response in the patient. Figure 2.11 shows the various reflected areas in the hand.

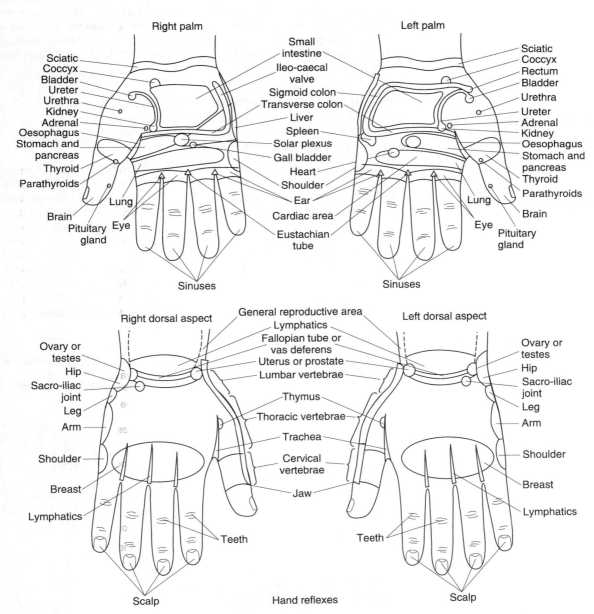

Figure 2.11 Reflexes of the hand.

(e) Meridian end points

Palpating the Tsing (end) points on the meridians correctly indicates the energetic quantity in that particular meridian. It is an easy procedure and can prove to be very useful. The patient just needs their hands and feet exposed as all the Tsing points lie on the sides of the nails of the fingers and toes. Please note that although these points may be useful in treatment as well as analysis, they do not represent *the* most powerful and effective points available, so the treatment capabilities of these points are limited. There is no particular 'batting' order in using these analytical points, but for simplicity's sake, it is usually better to start with the finger points followed by the foot ones. They are all 'nail' points with the exception of Kidney 1 which is situated on the sole of the foot in the midline, one-third down from the tip of the middle toe and two-thirds up from the heel base (Figure 2.12 highlights them):

Lung – Lu 11 (lateral aspect of the thumb)
Large intestine – LI 1 (lateral aspect of the forefinger)
Pericardium – P 9 (lateral aspect of the middle finger)
Triple heater – TH 1 (medial aspect of the ring finger)
Heart – Ht 9 (medial aspect of the little finger)
Small intestine – Si 1 (lateral aspect of the little finger)

Figure 2.12 Meridian end ponts.

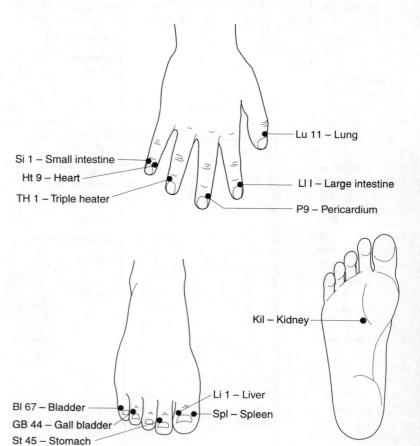

Kidney – Ki 1 (sole of the foot)
Spleen – Sp 1 (medial aspect of the great toe)
Liver – Li 1 (lateral aspect of the great toe)
Stomach – St 45 (lateral aspect of the second toe)
Gall bladder – GB 44 (lateral aspect of the fourth toe)
Bladder – Bl 67 (lateral aspect of the little toe)

Please note that there are no meridians on the middle toe. If the reader has not already studied acupuncture or shiatsu in detail, it may seem rather daunting at first to study all 12 points, but there is no substitute for painstaking study in order to learn them all. As mentioned before, they are not the most used meridian points in acupressure, but they are used on a regular basis, and of course are very useful in analysis. The technique is simple – gently palpate each Tsing point and give a short clockwise massage to each. Each and every acupoint, being a reflected point of an organ or system, should exhibit some degree of tenderness when palpated, so it is quite normal that the patient will feel them when these points are massaged. It is the actual sensation, though, that is important. If the patient feels acute discomfort almost to the point of being uncomfortable, this indicates that there is adequate energy, or even a Yang situation with too much energy in the meridian. If, however, on palpation and massage there is very little or no response from the patient, this will indicate that there is very little energy within the meridian, i.e. a Yin situation. Write all this information down and refer to it when you are ready to proceed to treatment. There are different techniques of treatment for acute and chronic conditions.

(f) Listening posts

The topic of 'listening posts' was introduced in the last book and brought about much discussion and intrigue from those who had not heard of it before. Since publication, I have spent much time in workshops teaching the various listening post procedures, so because it is an important topic, it will be discussed fully here. The term 'listening post' is derived from craniosacral therapy philosophy, and is used to ascertain the quality and quantity of cerebrospinal and interstitial fluid in a given system of the body, e.g. spine, soft tissue, joints etc. The usual areas of the body that are used as listening posts in craniosacral therapy are the occiput (cranial base), the sacrum and the heels. Craniosacral therapy practitioners and cranial osteopaths are taught to place both hands on the occiput (known as the vault hold) or the sacrum/heels and to 'tune in' to the flow of cerebrospinal fluid or energy flow. The author learnt this technique several years ago and has since adapted it by using isolated acupoints on the skull as listening posts to ascertain the energy quality and quantity in various systems of the body – for example, the endocrine glands, bony structures etc. The methods that will be discussed here will be the use of the vault hold for general analysis and the use of St 2, Extra 2, TH 17, LI 20, Bl 2 and Gov 16 with Extra 1 for individual system analysis. The sacrum is purposely not discussed because its use in analysis and treatment will be mentioned fully in other books in the series. Also not mentioned in this chapter are points GB 7 and St 8 (mentioned in the previous book) and Si 19 with GB 14, which will be discussed in the chapter on stress. The heel is also discussed in Chapter 6.

Up to this part of the book, the way the therapist 'feels' has generally been described as one where the patient exhibits some degree of discomfort when the therapist presses or massages the acupoint, thus indicating an imbalance in the point and hence underlying meridian or organ. With listening posts philosophy, the therapist 'tunes in' to the patient's energy flow of the whole body or a specific organ or system. A harmony is produced between the therapist and patient when both of them have a brain wave frequency of 7–8 Hz. Research has shown that the brain wave frequency where 'healing' and harmony occurs is the alpha–theta rhythm – around 8 Hz. True healing and one-ness cannot take place until this state of harmony is achieved. This statement is so important that it is going to be repeated – *True healing and one-ness cannot take place until this state of harmony is achieved*. At this frequency, both 'healer' and 'healee' (patient/client) are in a state of relaxation. In practical acupressure terms, the sensation that is felt is quite marked (even taking into account the subtlety of what is happening). There appears to be a 'shift' of sensation under the fingers – this is usually a lovely gentle warmth where none was before. Often, though not always, the patient also feels the shift of energy emphasis at the same time. This begins the time of one-ness between the therapist and the patient, and it is essential that this state of awareness is reached, especially when treating chronic conditions, before healing can take place. The phrase 'shift of energy emphasis' will be used several times in this book. This is where both therapist and patient attune together at around 8 Hz.

When using any of the listening posts mentioned, it is essential that the practitioner is relaxed with the arms supported as much as possible. It is possible that some of the holds will last for up to 10 minutes and the worst thing that can happen is for the arms and hands to become tired, cramped or go into a state of clonus – that can be very embarrassing for both patient and practitioner. The patient, too, should be in a state of relaxation, with the head well supported and *warm*. When using the vault hold, most therapists prefer to have an ordinary pillow placed under the patient's head. I prefer to use a small linen bag filled with small polystyrene balls, wheat germ or budgerigar seed. The therapist's hands can be glided easily underneath the cranial base and if there is any mobilizing or massage treatment to be done, it is easy to achieve this with the space and freedom of movement that is needed for these, plus having the patient's head supported at the same time. It is difficult to achieve this with an ordinary pillow. There are some purpose-made orthopaedic pillows on the market that also seem to fit the bill.

As has been stated before, this approach to the patient's energy analysis is much more than merely palpating and awaiting the grimaces on their face. There is interplay and union of the two energy systems. As such, the therapist has to be fully relaxed and yet have utmost concentration at all times. The use of thought is paramount in the interplay and because thoughts can be persuasive as well as 'powerful' there is a need to stay focused on the job in hand. Using listening posts employs the phenomenon of 'body dowsing'. This may, to the more orthodox practitioner, appear to be slightly esoteric, but having used these methods and techniques for several years now, it is second nature to me and seems a very natural thing to do. Dowsing is just another approach to analysing something and the practitioner is simply 'tuning in' to what the patient is attempting to express. The use of body dowsing is far more commonly practised than is imagined. It is used often in healing, reflexology, reiki and several other disciplines, sometimes without even the therapist realizing it. It is such a natural thing to attempt to tune in to what the patient is expressing that it is often taken for granted. Often there is no need for them to undress, and they will be warmer and more comfortable if they are allowed to keep their clothes on.

Vault hold

The patient lies in a supine position with their head supported, as previously mentioned, on some type of firm and supportive cushion. The therapist's hands are placed under the patients occiput, with the little fingers almost touching each other and the other fingers fairly close to each other (see Figure 2.13). Therapists who are well versed in craniosacral therapy will be used to this position; to the remainder of you, imagine that you are just cuddling and supporting the back of the head. It is also important that the forearms and elbows are supported on the couch, otherwise fatigue will soon set in. The contact must be very light and 'airy' with no pressure whatsoever placed upon the patient's skull (slightly different with cranial osteopathy!). Nothing will happen for approximately 30 seconds to a minute, so patience is required. After this time it is quite

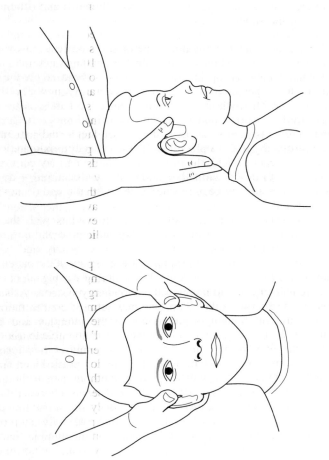

Figure 2.13 Vault hold.

natural that a certain amount of warmth will be created under the hands, this is merely body heat. Also at this time it is perfectly natural for the patient to wriggle and squirm a little as they start to assume a more relaxed and comfortable position. Never be in a hurry for things to start happening and *never* try and speed things on. Patients react at their own speed and each person is different. After approximately 1–2 minutes the therapist should start to feel the 'cranial rhythm'. This is a naturally occurring rhythm of the cerebrospinal fluid flow. Some schools of thought insist that this rhythm represents the actual cerebrospinal flow in a physical way, others insist that it is really an interpretation of it – more on the lines of a holographic image, whilst others say it is merely the body's vital force that is perceived. I do not intend to enter any debate here as to which one I feel is correct. Students of mine will know which is my preference, but it does not mean to say that it is correct. The sensations that are felt may be interpreted in the way the practitioner wishes to interpret them – it does not matter! The cranial rhythm ranges in individuals between 6 and 20 cycles per minute. The sensations felt under the hands are like a subtle expansion and contraction. One cycle is the time taken from the beginning of the expansion phase to the start of the next one. This energetic sensation can also be likened to the movement of the tide on the beach – it is in constant flow. It is too crude to call the rhythm 'in–out', as some colleges teach. The phases of the cranial flow should, more properly, be called 'expansion' and 'contraction'; this is a good name for it especially when explaining what is happening to the subtle energy in a clinical way, but even this definition does not do it justice.

It is important that the rhythm is perceived and held for at least 2 minutes whilst at the same time keeping the 'brain in neutral', in other words try not to have any specific thoughts in your head except the ones of concentration on perceiving the cranial rhythm. By now the therapist should feel a warm rhythmical pulsation under the hands. After a short time, a definite shift of emphasis will be perceived under the hands. As explained previously, this is where the practitioner's and patient's vital force are resonating in the alpha–theta frequency at approximately 8 c.p.s. Once this has been reached, the task of body dowsing may commence. It is not possible to dowse until the 'tuning in' has occurred – do not be fooled that it has already been reached when it hasn't, and do not try and speed things on.

The next phase of analysis using the vault hold is with the use of thought. It is my belief that thought is very influential and can be quite powerful and manipulative, so it is to be used wisely and with due deference to the task in hand. 'Questions' are asked about the patient's vital force and energy flow (or cerebrospinal fluid flow) by using silent thought. On no account is the therapist to speak out loud or to obviously change the position of the hands in any way that may suggest to the patient that something different is taking place. The answers to the questions that are asked have to be in the positive or negative, it is impossible to ask obscure questions that give 'woolly' answers. The vault hold is used for general energy questions and the specific acupoints that are detailed later deal with individual energy systems. If the answer to a question is in the negative (patient's energy system says 'No'), the rhythm that is felt under the hands continues unabated. If the answer to the question is in the positive (patient's energy system says 'Yes'), the rhythm appears to stop or to go into a continuous contraction phase. It is vital that the mind is cleared and the rhythm resumes before the next question is asked. Try not to be in a hurry, although it is a great temptation to do so with those therapists who may be practising this technique for the first time. It is extremely important that the therapist appreciates that this technique should only be used in the analysis of the patient's energy system at the moment of the procedure. It *cannot* be used to ask questions that deal with past or future conditions. Please be aware that it is a privilege to use this system; it can be very accurate and powerful but it should not be abused. An example of the type of question that can be asked would be 'Is there a deficiency of energy in the Lung meridian?'. If the answer to that particular question is 'Yes', the rhythm will seemingly stop or appear to be in a contraction phase. If the answer to the question is 'No', the rhythm will stay the same. Clear the mind and allow a couple of rhythmical cycles before attempting to ask the next question. As stated before, the vault hold may be used with general energy questions or to ascertain the state of the cerebrospinal fluid flow or indeed, with practice, to ask any question at all. It may also be used in treatment mode, but that is outside the scope of this book. It will, however, be discussed in the book on 'Healing with the Chakra Energy System'.

Specific cranial acupoints used as listening posts

I have used the vault hold, heels and sacrum holds as listening posts for several years and have had excellent results with both patients and delegates alike. About 10 years ago I started to experiment in using individual cranial acupoints to ascertain the energetic flow in specific systems. There are points that can be used specifically in musculo-skeletal, endocrine, digestive, eliminative, urinary, circulatory, respiratory, emotional and neural systems. Figure 2.14 shows the main points that can be used, although it is not exhaustive. Points St 8 (soft tissue energy) and GB 7 (muscle and tendon energy) were discussed in the last book whilst Si 19 (temporo-mandibular joint (TMJ) and emotional energy) and GB 14 (emotional energy) will be discussed in the chapter on stress release.

Method

The patient lies supine with the head comfortable on a suitable pillow and the therapist sits behind the patient's head and slowly introduces the pads of the middle fingers to the various points described below. Make sure that the forearms are well supported on the couch. All the points used are bilateral ones, hence the left middle finger is placed on the left side of the patient's head and the right finger on their right side. Just as with the vault hold, and indeed any prolonged point hold, after a couple of minutes the emphasis of touch changes into an easier, harmonious feeling. Nothing else will happen until this shift of emphasis has taken place. After this change, the practitioner has to concentrate on the aspect of the patient's energy system that is under analysis. This method of energy analysis is often called 'finger dowsing' and is something that may not 'click' with therapists straight away; it takes time to master. As in the vault hold analysis above, the therapist simply 'asks questions' of the patient's energy system and it is done purely by concentrated thought and not aloud. What usually occurs with this procedure is that the sensations under the fingers change as the questions change. There appears to be a 'stillness' of movement in chronic conditions, and much heat and 'activity' in acute conditions. It is always best to ascertain the overall energy picture of the

Figure 2.14 Listening posts.

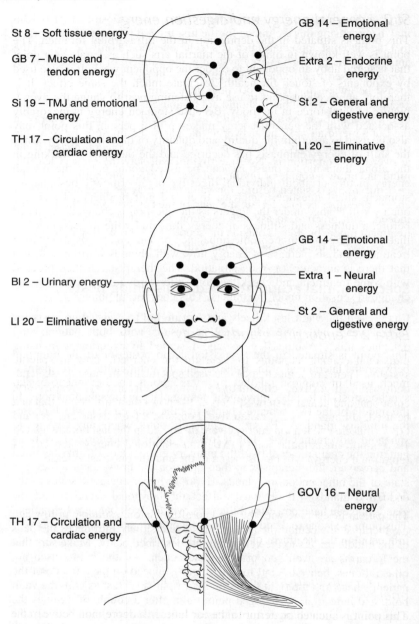

St 8 – Soft tissue energy

GB 7 – Muscle and tendon energy

Si 19 – TMJ and emotional energy

TH 17 – Circulation and cardiac energy

GB 14 – Emotional energy

Extra 2 – Endocrine energy

St 2 – General and digestive energy

LI 20 – Eliminative energy

Bl 2 – Urinary energy

LI 20 – Eliminative energy

GB 14 – Emotional energy

Extra 1 – Neural energy

St 2 – General and digestive energy

GOV 16 – Neural energy

TH 17 – Circulation and cardiac energy

system first before proceeding to ask specific questions about individual 'parts' of the body. The points need only be held until the change of emphasis has occurred and the therapist is satisfied that the information being gleaned is constant and correct. Prolonged holding of the points enable them to be used in treatment mode. This is achieved by keeping the fingers *in situ*, concentrating totally on the system or body part that is in a state of imbalance, gently twisting and turning to the movement of the energy flow whilst keeping the fingers on the points. This procedure is quite advanced and it is recommended that it is only attempted by experienced practitioners.

St 2 – general energy and digestion energy

This point is situated in the depression in the infra-orbital foramen. The point is well known in many of the martial arts such as karate as a point that is stared at by an opponent to render the opponent weak. It is also used by exponents of 'touch for health' to create much the same effect. It is therefore an excellent point to use as a listening post to gauge the overall picture of vital force in the body. Because stomach energy is inexorably associated with the general energy make-up of a person, this point may also be used to ascertain the quality and quantity of digestive energy. Once the shift of energy emphasis has occurred and the therapist is working in the alpha–theta mode, questions can be asked about either the overall energy picture or about individual digestive organs (mouth, oesophagus, stomach, small intestine, pancreas, liver and gall bladder). The energy quality will change under the fingers as the question is changed. As stated before, a dullness and stillness of energy flow under the fingers indicates that the body part is in a chronic imbalance or Yin, and needs stimulating treatment, and an increase of energy flow with obvious warmth indicates that there is an acute, or Yang situation. The therapist can then proceed with some treatment and check the point afterwards to see if there is any change in sensation under the fingers. This goes for all points.

Extra 2 – endocrine glands energy

This point is situated in the depression 1 cun posterior to the midpoint between the lateral end of the eyebrow and the outer canthus. This point is much used in craniosacral therapy as the point on the spheno-basilar synchondrosis to feel the 'movement' taking place in the sphenoid bone. In the middle of the two sphenoid bones lies the sella tursica, which houses the pituitary gland. As Extra 2 is the only point where any changes in sphenoid movement can be felt, it follows that it is of enormous value in gauging the energetic quality of the pituitary gland. Once this has been felt and perceived, the therapist can then question the body about the energy state of the other endocrine glands. Hypo- or hyper-energetic states of the endocrine glands will obviously affect the hormonal secretions of the glands and can have powerful influences over the well being of the patient. This point is also associated with the brow or third eye chakra, so it is very influential in the treatment of pituitary dysfunction.

TH 17 – circulation energy, heat energy and cardiac energy

This point is situated posterior to the ear lobe, in a depression between the angle of the mandible and the mastoid process. This is a very influential point. It is said to be the ear chakra (one of the minor chakras) which in turn is related to the heart chakra; it is therefore vital in the analysis and treatment of circulatory and cardiac conditions. It is also said to be directly linked to the hypothalamus via the internal meridian system. The hypothalamus, amongst many other functions, deals with the heating mechanism of the body. When used as a listening post, TH 17 can gauge the well being or otherwise of the blood circulation (arterial and venous) and also the lymphatic circulation. It is also, by questioning, able to give guidelines as to the cause of hot and cold conditions such as cold hands and feet. It is a very versatile point.

LI 20 – respiratory energy and large bowel (eliminative) energy

This point is situated between the naso-labial groove and the midpoint of the outer point of the nasal ala. It is the last point on the large intestine meridian and is very influential in treatment mode in sinusitis, catarrh, some skin conditions and large bowel imbalance. The large bowel meridian is closely tied in with the lung meridian in that they are both associated with excretion and the eliminative system – they form the duo of organs in the 'metal' element (see Chapter 3). It is therefore the ideal point to be used as a listening post in the analysis of respiratory and excretory conditions. Start questioning on a broad basis firstly and gradually narrow it down to specific areas of the body that may be of concern. This advice is true for all points, but it is amazing how this basic precept is ignored by therapists – they want to get to the root of the problem as quickly as possible. This is an understandable situation, we all want to do things as quickly as possible, but if this procedure of starting broadly and narrowing down the questioning is not carried out, it is possible that much vital information could be missed. *Never* assume the answers in advance; there are often exciting surprises to be had.

Bl 2 – Urinary energy and sexual energy

This point is situated in the depression proximal to the medial end of the eyebrow, directly above the inner canthus. As it lies on the bladder meridian, the point can be used as a listening post for all urinary conditions both acute and chronic, such as cystitis, prostatitis and nephritis. The point is also very close to Extra 1 (brow chakra), which has links, amongst others, with the reproductive system, so it seems to be the perfect point in the analysis of conditions of internal organs within the pelvis. Please note that it should not be used in hormonal imbalances to do with the testes and uterus; the best point for that is Extra 2 as previously described.

Gov 16 with Extra 1 – neural energy

The last individual listening post to be discussed is the most unusual one and perhaps the most far reaching. It is unusual in that two different points are used. Although the points are not bilateral ones on the same meridian, they are integrally linked with each other as being the anterior and posterior aspects of the brow (Ajna) chakra and as such are very powerful and influential points when used as a duo. The full diagnostic and treatment capabilities of these two points would take several pages to explain, but will be fully discussed in the book that deals with the chakra energy system.

Gov 16 is situated directly below the occipital protuberance, in the midline, in a large depression. Extra 1 is situated between the medial end of the two eyebrows and is often called the glabella. It is important that the therapist should be comfortable with the forearms supported and that the patient's head is kept as straight as possible with the face uppermost. It is a temptation to turn their head when locating these two points and not return it to the upright position! It is also a temptation to rest the middle finger that is in contact with Extra 1 a little too heavily; remember that light and subtle touch only is needed – any added pressure will negate the responses. Although these two points can have wide-ranging analytical and treatment uses, it is the perfect listening post for conditions associated with central nervous system imbalance. These can include any neurological condition, conditions of the spinal cord, peripheral motor and sensory nerves and also questions about the autonomic nervous system. Because of the length of time that the fingers need to be held *in situ* with these two points once the shift of emphasis has taken place, it is more than likely that the treatment mode will also be activated. There is no need to worry about this. These two points are used extensively in stress release and in such conditions as anxiety control, so the only side effect is that the patient may become so relaxed that they may fall asleep. The energy system is still receptive during sleep, in fact experience has shown that the energy systems can be analysed and treated far quicker. The downside of the patient falling asleep is that they may produce the kind of noises from their mouths and nostrils that are usually associated with night-time slumber. Snoring can become quite a problem and it is often better to gently wake them. It should be recognized as a privilege, though, that the patient has so much confidence in you that they submit to slumber.

3

Meridians, acupoints and reflexes

Meridians are the invisible vessels in traditional Chinese medicine (TCM) that 'house' the body's vital force or Chi. As has already been mentioned, there are 12 bilateral meridians, each being related to and associated with an internal organ. There are also two unilateral meridians and six others that are composites of the main ones. Table 3.1 shows the 12 bilateral meridians and their relationships, while Table 3.2 shows the important points that are of use in acupressure.

Looking at Table 3.1, it can be seen that energy flows in a logical sequence from organ/meridian to organ/meridian. For example, with the arms outstretched above the head, Yin energy flows upwards and Yang energy flows downwards. This knowledge is very important, as the actual direction of energy flow makes all the difference in the different acupressure techniques, especially meridian massage.

Yang meridians tend to lie on the posterior and lateral aspects of the limbs, whereas Yin meridians lie on the anterior and medial aspects. In a way, it seems that the Yin energy is protected and the Yang energy is open, thus mimicking the organs themselves. On each meridian there are a few

Table 3.1 The 12 bilateral meridians and their relationships

'Peak' time	Meridian	Yin/Yang	Element	Direction of energy flow
0300	Lung	Yin	Metal	Chest to hand
0500	Large intestine	Yang	Metal	Hand to face
0700	Stomach	Yang	Earth	Face to foot
0900	Spleen	Yin	Earth	Foot to chest
1100	Heart	Yin	Fire	Chest to hand
1300	Small intestine	Yang	Fire	Hand to face
1500	Bladder	Yang	Water	Face to foot
1700	Kidney	Yin	Water	Foot to chest
1900	Pericardium	Yin	Fire	Chest to hand
2100	Three heater	Yang	Fire	Hand to face
2300	Gall bladder	Yang	Wood	Face to foot
0100	Liver	Yin	Wood	Foot to chest

Table 3.2 Important points on the meridian

Meridian	Symbol	From	To	No. of points	Source	Tonification	Great	Type
Stomach	St	Eye	Second toe	45	42	41	36	Yang
Spleen	Sp	Great toe	Sixth intercostal space	21	3	2	6	Yin
Heart	Ht	Axilla	Little finger	9	7	9	7	Yin
Small intestine	Si	Little finger	Ear	19	4	3	3	Yang
Bladder	Bl	Eye	Little toe	67	64	67	62	Yang
Kidney	Ki	Sole of foot	Clavicle	27	3	7	6	Yin
Pericardium	P	Chest	Middle finger	9	7	9	6	Yin
Three heater	TH	Ring finger	Ear	23	4	3	5	Yang
Gall bladder	GB	Eye	Fourth toe	44	40	43	41	Yang
Liver	Li	Great toe	Chest	11	3	8	3	Yin
Lung	Lu	Chest	Thumb	11	9	9	7	Yin
Large intestine	LI	Index finger	Nose	20	4	11	4	Yang

points described that are particularly significant in acupressure therapy. They are the *Tsing* or nail point, the *source* point, the *tonification* point and the *great* point. Occasionally these overlap – it will be pointed out where they do.

The *Tsing* or nail points, being at the start or end of a meridian, vary in importance in each meridian. They are always situated at the side of a nail and are usually painful when pressed. When they are not mentioned in the text, they have no importance in acupressure therapy.

The *source* points are those points on the meridian that most easily affects the actual organs associated with the meridians. In other words, they represent a short cut of energy boosting to the organ. These points are the second most important points on each meridian.

The *tonification* points are those points where energy can be 'transferred' from one meridian to another, thus creating a balance of energy. This is achieved by balancing energy around the Sheng cycle as in the law of five elements. This technique is discussed in Chapter 5.

The *great* points are the most important points on the meridians in that they have more than one function. They are usually the most 'powerful' point on the meridian, being used more than any other points in meridian acupressure. If readers wish to memorize the great points, they will go a long way to being able to practice clinical acupressure successfully.

Meridians and acupoints

Stomach meridian

This meridian starts just below the eyeball. It then descends to the mandible, loops up to the hairline, passing over the temporomandibular joint, re-emerging half way down the antero-lateral aspect of the neck. It then travels following a line through the nipple 4 cun lateral to the midline through the groin. It re-emerges on the anterior aspect of the upper thigh

Figure 3.1 Stomach meridian.

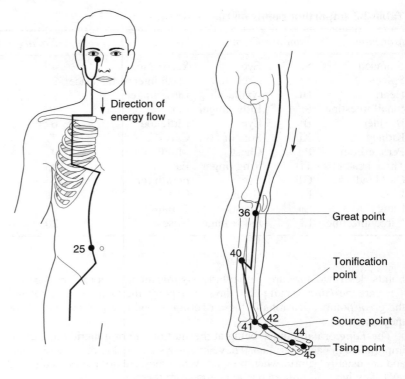

descending to the lateral nail point of the second toes. It is unique in that it is the only Yang meridian that is situated on the anterior aspect of the torso chest and abdomen (Figure 3.1).

Associations

Energy type – Yang
Energy peak time – 0700 hrs
No. of points – 45
Element – Earth
Yin pairing – spleen
Sense – taste
System – connective tissue
Sense organ – mouth
Colour – yellow
Season – late summer
Taste – sweet
Weather – humidity
Emotional – depression, anxiety

The stomach has the function of receiving food (energy), separating out the pure essence that it passes on to the spleen and impure (waste) that it passes on to the small intestine for eventual secretion. The natural function of the stomach is to send Chi downward for further processing. If this function is in any way impaired, then the stomach Chi is said to 'rebelling upwards'. This leads to belching, hiccups, regurgitation, nausea and vomiting. It goes without saying that in order to maintain a good energy balance within the stomach, a person's eating habits need to be sound. In attempting to remedy many stomach and general energy imbalances, it is often sufficient to indicate to the patient that a good balanced diet is required. The stomach meridian is also useful in the treatment of some emotional imbalances. The points and methods will be highlighted in Chapter 6.

Source point – St 42

Situated 1.5 cun distal to St 41 at the highest part of the dorsum of the foot. The main action is to relieve stomach ache by gently stimulating the point for a few seconds, then sedating it for up to 5 minutes or until such time as the pain eases.

Tonification point – St 41

Situated on the mid-point of the dorsum of the foot on the ankle joint between the tendons of extensor digitorum and hallucis longus. This point is used in transfer of energy via the Sheng cycle to the large intestine meridian.

Great point – St 36

This point lies one finger's breadth from the anterior crest of the tibia, between it and the fibula, and 3 cun below the inferior and lateral aspect of the patella.

Uses:

1. General tonification of energy of the body by stimulating massage.
2. Any upper gastrointestinal tract imbalance, e.g. nausea, vomiting, gastralgia. To make someone vomit the contents of the stomach, heavy stimulation is needed. To calm down gastralgia, light massage or gentle sedation is required.
3. Migraine, especially when pain settles over one eye and the cause can be attributed to the eating of a migraine 'trigger' food, e.g. cheese or chocolate.
4. Vagus nerve imbalance, i.e. vertigo or dizziness. It also helps clear a 'woolly' head or 'brain fog'.
5. Upper palate toothache. Use just sedation here.

This represents one of the very great points in acupressure. It is probably the best point on the body for 'energy giving'. When there is low vitality both physically and mentally, St 36 should be stimulated quite aggressively for up to 5 minutes. This can be done bilaterally at the same time. The only exception to this is in the very young (babies and small children). It works wonders in the elderly!

Contra-indications: Do not perform stimulating massage after the patient has had a heavy meal or if they already have nausea. In these instances, sedation is required. Also contra-indicated in cases of stomach cancer.

Spleen meridian

The spleen meridian commences at the medial nail point of the great toe, passes along the medial border of the foot and ascends the medial aspect

Figure 3.2 Spleen meridian.

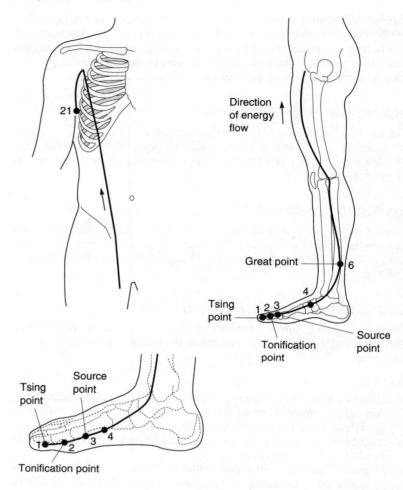

of the leg to the medial area below the knee joint. It then ascends the anterior aspect of the thigh and emerges in the abdomen 4 cun lateral to the midline. It then passes up to the second intercostal space and descends to finish in the sixth intercostal space in the mid-axillary line (Figure 3.2).

Associations

Energy type – Yin
Energy peak time – 0900 hrs
No. of points – 21
Element – Earth
Yang pairing – stomach
Sense – taste
System – connective tissue
Sense organ – mouth
Colour – yellow
Season – late summer
Taste – sweet

Weather – humidity
Emotional – depression, rage

The spleen has much more importance in TCM than it has in orthodox medicine. It is seen as the primary organ of digestion. The spleen extracts the nutrients from food in the stomach which forms the basis of Chi and blood, and transports it to the heart and lungs. A healthy spleen will mean a good appetite, digestion, energy and muscle tone. When it is imbalanced, this will lead to fatigue, abdominal distension, poor digestion and diarrhoea. Sluggishness of energy flow in the spleen is also associated with the accumulation of body fluids which can lead to 'internal damp' conditions such as oedema and obesity. The spleen is also said to be involved with the immune system. Stimulation of spleen points can help restore the body's immune strength and fight off invading micro-organisms. The spleen is also said to be associated with blood Chi, and impaired energy flow can lead to varicosities and haemorrhoids. The spleen meridian is also used in many gynaecological disorders which may or may not be due to 'stuck blood' conditions as in amenorrhoea. On an emotional level, the spleen has the role of sending clear energy to the head and brain. This results in clarity of thought that can give the sense of lightness and well being. When the spleen is impaired there will be a deficiency of clear energy reaching the head, which can result in muzzy and disordered thinking, leading to lethargy and fatigue.

Source point – Sp 3

This point is situated posterior and inferior to the head of the first metacarpal. It is particularly used in treating gastralgia, diarrhoea, vomiting and constipation. Stimulate for diarrhoea and sedate in constipation.

Tonification point – Sp 2

This point is situated on the medial aspect of the Gt toe, anterior and inferior to the first metatarso-phalangeal (MTP) joint. As well as treating abdominal distension, it is used to regulate energy flow along with the lung meridian.

Great point – Sp 6

This point is situated 3 cun superior to the medial malleolus just posterior to the tibial border.

Uses:

1. Restoration of energy in cases of general weakness.
2. Gastro-intestinal conditions.
3. Internal inflammations and ulcerations of the uterus and ovaries.
4. Intra-uterine bleeding and bleeding haemorrhoids.
5. Anaesthesia – general point.
6. Gravitational ulcer – parallel point.

Sp 6 is simply *the* great point in uterine conditions. Its anaesthetic qualities are best enhanced if used in conjunction with LI 4. It is very useful in period pain and also in permitting an easier childbirth. In conjunction with

St 36 it is used in restoring vitality in cases of generalized weakness. Stimulating massage is needed for this.

Other useful spleen points

Sp 4 is located on the medial aspect of the foot in a depression at the anterior and inferior border of the first metatarsal bone. It is one of the *key points* of the eight extraordinary meridians, and has the general use of easing feelings of suffocation and stuffiness. It can also be used as a revival point, and is applied as such in certain martial arts.

Sp 21 is situated on the mid axillary line in the sixth intercostal space. It is used locally for chest pains and other localized pain. Generally, it is considered to be the intercostal chakra and, although it is a minor chakra, it is a significantly powerful point, being useful as an adjunct point in the treatment of low blood pressure, chronic respiratory conditions and anything where there are 'bony' abnormalities due to an imbalance of calcium formation, e.g. Scheurmann's disease and ankylosing spondylitis. (Explanations of how these points can be used to treat chronic conditions such as those mentioned will be given in Chapter 5.)

Heart meridian

The heart meridian is the shortest of all the meridians. The first point is in the axilla, and the meridian descends the antero-medial arm and forearm, crossing the palm and ending at the nail point on the lateral side of the little finger (Figure 3.3).

Associations

Energy type – Yin
Energy peak time – 1100 hrs
No. of points – 9
Element – Fire
Yang pairing – small intestine
Sense – speech
System – circulation
Sense organ – tongue
Colour – red
Season – summer
Taste – bitter
Weather – heat
Emotion – excess joy, euphoria

In TCM the function of the heart is close to the conventional Western view. The heart controls and regulates the flow of blood through the body. This is essential to ensure a healthy supply of blood to all the tissues. A healthy functioning heart will result in an even warmth in the extremities of the body and a regular and even pulse. Impaired functioning may lead to cold extremities and the classical heart-related chest pains. The blood vessels are seen to be an extension of the heart. Good functioning will lead to a healthy circulation whilst impaired function may give arterial sclerosis etc. It is said that the tongue is the mirror of the heart, although the condition

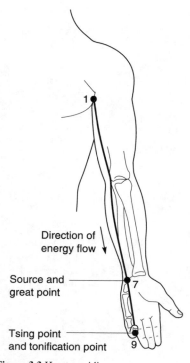

Direction of energy flow

Source and great point

7

Tsing point and tonification point

9

Figure 3.3 Heart meridian.

of other organs can be gauged from the tongue, it is the heart function that most readily shows in the tongue, especially at the tip. It is, though, the emotions and psyche that are most governed by the heart meridian. The myriad of mental, psychological and spiritual faculties are grouped together in one word in TCM – Shen. It is probably best described as the force that shapes the personality. When the heart has Shen under control, we are at peace with the world and our surroundings. If the heart energy is in a state of imbalance, this can lead to a whole range of mental and psychological disorders. The main emotion that is associated with the heart is joy. It will be pointed out in Chapter 6 how many stress-related conditions may be treated with the heart and associated energy channels.

Tsing point and tonification point – Ht 9

This point is situated on the radial side of the little finger as the nail point. It is useful in the treatment of chest pains and acute situations involving the heart, as well as the point used on the Yin Sheng cycle of the five elements in passing on energy to the spleen meridian.

Source point and great point – Ht 7

This point is located on the ulnar side of the wrist crease just proximal to the pisiform bone.

Uses:

1. Nervous anxiety such as stage fright or examination nerves.
2. Sleeplessness due to anxiety or stress. Strong rhythmical massage is needed here, maybe combined with a little sheep counting and preceded by a couple of herbal valerian tablets.
3. Emotional trauma. One of the best uses of this point that is not mentioned in other texts, but seems to work, is that of emotional 'blockage' removal – as in bottling of emotions after a death in the family or similar emotional trauma. The heart meridian tends to 'soak up' this tension. It is excellent when combined with LI 4.
4. Local use in wrist pain and used as a distal point in axilla pain.

As the reader can see, the great point associated with the heart meridian Ht 7 (Shenmen) is one of the most powerful points in acupressure that lifts Shen and clears the mind. It is *the* best point in insomnia and anticipation. It is not by accident that it is given the same Chinese name as the point in the ear that is also related to calming Shen. Ear acupressure will be discussed later in this chapter.

Small intestine meridian

This channel starts at the lateral nail point of the little finger, passes upwards on the ulnar and dorsal aspect of the forearm and arm to the posterior aspect of the shoulder. It then goes on a zigzag course across the back of the shoulder and into the lateral aspect of the cervical spine to the cheek where it finishes anterior to the ear (Figure 3.4).

Figure 3.4 Small intestine meridian.

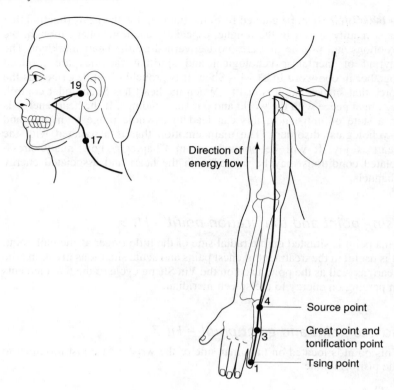

Direction of energy flow

Source point

Great point and tonification point

Tsing point

Associations

Energy type – Yang
Energy peak time – 1300 hrs
No. of points – 19
Element – Fire
Yin pairing – heart
Sense – speech
System – Circulation
Sense organ – tongue
Colour – red
Season – summer
Taste – bitter
Weather – heat
Emotional – excess joy

In TCM, the small intestine function does not really differ from the orthodox medicine viewpoint. It receives partially digested food from the stomach. The pure is extracted under the control of the spleen, and the impure is then passed either to the large intestine or to the bladder for excretion. It can easily be affected by the type and temperature of food eaten. Too much cold and raw food can create cold in the small bowel, whilst excess of hot foods can create heat. It is also considered to be the organ of assimilation, where 'sorting out' takes place. This occurs on an emotional as well as physical level.

Source point – Si 4

This point is situated at the ulnar side of the border of the palm in the depression by the proximal end of the fifth metacarpal bone. It is a useful point in vomiting and tinnitus.

Tonification point and great point – Si 3

This point is situated proximal to the fifth metacarpo-phalangeal joint on the ulnar border of the hand.

Uses:

1. Diarrhoea – use stimulation here.
2. Constipation – use gentle massage over a long period (at least 5 minutes).
3. Posterior shoulder pain, trigeminal neuralgia and elbow pain.
4. It is one of the key points of the eight extraordinary meridians (governor channel), forming a couple with Bl 62. Because of this association, it is used in the treatment of many painful spinal conditions.
5. Used as an emergency point (with LI 2) in the treatment of nose bleeds (epistaxis).

Bladder meridian

The bladder meridian is the longest meridian, with 67 points. It starts at the inner canthus of the eye, ascends the forehead and passes over the frontal bone and down to the occiput 0.5 cun from the midline. It then divides into two branches. The more medial branch descends from the level of T2 down to S4 1.5 cun lateral to the midline. The outer branch descends from T2 to S4 3 cun lateral to the midline. The inner branch ascends from S4 to the first sacral foramen and descends again to 0.5 cun lateral to the coccyx. It re-emerges at the mid point of the gluteal fold and passes down the posterior aspect of the thigh to the mid-point of the popliteal fossa where it joins again with the lateral branch. The combined meridian then descends between the lateral and medial bellies of the gastrocnemius muscle, tracks lateral to the midline of the leg, passing inferior to the lateral malleolus along the lateral border of the foot, to terminate at the nail point on the outer aspect of the little toe (Figure 3.5).

Associations

Energy type – Yang
Energy peak time – 1500 hrs
No. of points – 67
Element – Water
Yin pairing – kidney
Sense – hearing
System – bones
Sense organ – ears
Colour – black

Figure 3.5 Bladder meridian.

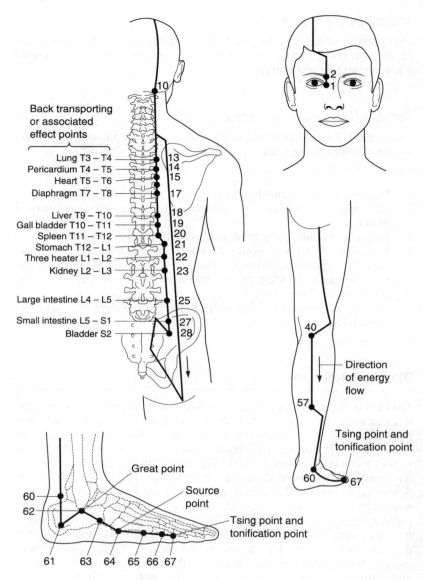

Back transporting
or associated
effect points

Lung T3 – T4
Pericardium T4 – T5
Heart T5 – T6
Diaphragm T7 – T8

Liver T9 – T10
Gall bladder T10 – T11
Spleen T11 – T12
Stomach T12 – L1
Three heater L1 – L2
Kidney L2 – L3

Large intestine L4 – L5

Small intestine L5 – S1
Bladder S2

Direction
of energy
flow

Tsing point and
tonification point

Great point

Source
point

Tsing point and
tonification point

Season – winter
Taste – salt
Weather – cold
Emotion – fear

The bladder meridian is perhaps the most used one when treating musculo-skeletal conditions, because of its course down the spine and leg. It is, though, used often in medical conditions, via the associated effect points that lie on the back. The bladder, of course, stores urine and controls excretion. It receives waste body fluids from the lungs, small intestine and large intestine and under the influence of the kidneys it stores and excretes this as urine. It is also a useful meridian when used in certain emotional conditions such as anxiety and fear.

Tsing point and tonification point – Bl 67

This nail point is situated on the lateral border of the little toe. This very painful point (pressure is not so painful as needle) has a particular use in painful labour in childbirth. In TCM, the point is given moxa for up to 5 days in cases of possible breach birth delivery. It is said that after this treatment the head engages normally. The author does not have any first-hand experience of using this point in this way, although anecdotally, colleagues have told me that they have found it extremely useful. The point needs to be stimulated for up to 5 minutes at a time with about an hour in between sessions. It is useful to combine this point with Sp 6. As the accumulation point it is used to pass energy on to the gall bladder meridian.

Source point – Bl 64

This point is situated below the tuberosity on the lateral aspect of the fifth metatarsal bone. It is indicated in the treatment of acute cystitis.

Great point – Bl 62

This point is located 0.5 cun directly below the lateral malleolus.

Uses:

1. Pain relief for such conditions as low back pain, sciatica, dorsal and cervical pain. It is one of the very great points in these cases.
2. It is one of the key points of the eight extraordinary meridians and is coupled with Si 3 in this capacity. It can be used by itself or in combination with Si 3 in the treatment of the pain in rheumatoid arthritis, osteoarthritis and spinal pain. It is also very useful in the treatment of autoimmune disorders.

Other useful bladder points

Bl 2 is situated directly above the inner canthus in a small hollow on the medial side of the brow. It has already been described as the listening post point associated with the urinary system. It is also very effective in the treatment of eye pain, frontal headaches, migraine and frontal sinusitis.

Bl 10 is situated 1.5 cun lateral to the midline at the C1–2 level. It is used in unison or with GB 20 in the treatment of occipital headaches. It is also very useful in clearing the head in stuffiness and when feeling dizzy and muzzy.

Bl 40 is located in the centre of the popliteal fossa. In acupressure, it is very useful as a distal point in spinal pain and lumbago. It is also useful as one of the many points that can be used in skin conditions.

Bl 66 is situated in the depression anterior and inferior to the fifth metatarso-phalangeal joint. Although it isn't the source point, it is said to have a stronger influence on easing conditions such as cystitis and lower abdominal pain than does Bl 64.

The *back transporting points* (*associated effect points*) that lie on the bladder line adjacent to the spine have a very important influence on the internal organs. It is thought that they have their influence via the chain of sympathetic (autonomic) nerves that lie adjacent to the spine. Although they are all meridian points, some texts place them as being reflex points of the spine. The author has no quarrel with this, it merely underlines the similarity between acupoints and reflexes. They lie on the inner bladder line (see Figure 3.5), which is 1.5 cun lateral to the spinous processes. They become tender when the associated organ is in a state of stress (Yin or Yang). The more Yang or acutely sick the organ, the more tender the point. They can be of use in two different ways:

1. As reflex points (diagnostic or treatment) to help support the energetic quality and quantity of the underlying organ. For example, Bl 23 (which is 1.5 cun lateral to the space between the spinous processes of L2–L3) is associated with the kidneys. The points will be tender if there is any acute kidney imbalance, or if there is any imbalance with the adrenal glands. It will also be tender to a deeper palpation with chronic kidney imbalances as in chronic nephritis or osteoarthritis. The usual rules of acupressure apply – sedate for the acute and stimulate for the chronic.
2. They can also be used as local points in the treatment of spinal conditions. This was described in the last book.

There are also some points on the outer bladder meridian that are associated with the underlying organs. Experience has shown that these points are useful in the treatment of emotional/mental conditions. These will be discussed in Chapter 6.

Kidney meridian

The kidney meridian originates on the sole of the foot, passes along the medial aspect of the ankle, circles the medial malleolus, and ascends the medial part of the leg to the knee. It then passes into the groin via the medial aspect of the thigh emerging 0.5 cun lateral to the midline and ascends the abdomen to the thorax where it is sited 2 cun from the midline and terminates just below the clavicle (Figure 3.6).

Associations

Energy type – Yin
Energy peak time – 1700 hrs
No. of points – 27
Element – Water
Yang pairing – bladder
Sense – hearing
System – bones
Sense organ – ears
Colour – black
Season – winter
Taste – salt
Weather – cold
Emotional – fear

It was mentioned in the previous chapter that every person inherits a certain constitutional energy from their parents and grandparents. This is called ancestral energy. It is said to be stored in the kidney meridians and organs. The kidneys therefore represent the 'deepest' of organs, and together with the heart, the maintenance of their energy is of the utmost importance. In TCM terminology, the ancestral energy is called 'Jing'. It is

Figure 3.6 Kidney meridian.

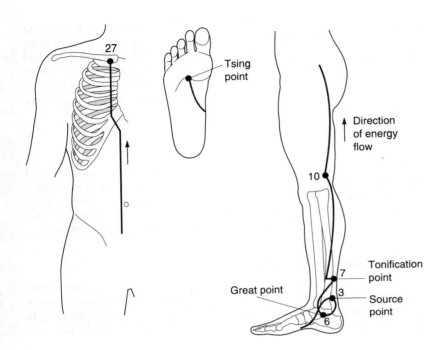

said to be the essence of life itself. It is partly inherited from our ancestors and partly extracted from food. Jing determines the constitutional strength and is an essential component of every aspect of the body. It is particularly the basis of growth and development through childhood and also fundamental to normal sexual and reproductive functioning throughout life.

When kidney energy is impaired in any way, often for constitutional reasons, this can lead to retarded growth, learning difficulties, infertility, sexual disorders or premature senility. Kidney energy is also essential for the formation of marrow, bones, teeth and an efficient brain function. When kidney energy is deficient it can lead to general coldness, lethargy and impaired sexual function (impotence or premature ejaculation for example). The kidneys also regulate the fluid balance in the body and their energy is essential in eliminating water from the body via urine or perspiration. The sense association is the ears and hearing. Deficiency in energy may lead to premature deafness or tinnitus. It is also said that the growth of hair also relies of kidney energy, although dull, lifeless and brittle hair may be caused by a number of factors. Kidney energy is also associated with the base emotion of fear. The kidneys are seen as the root of life, and thus the sense of personal power and will to succeed in life are rooted in healthy kidney functioning. Consequently, poor kidney functioning will lead to feelings of weakness and timidity – of being unable to face the demands made by life itself (Figure 3.6).

Tsing point – Ki 1

This is the only Tsing point that is not near a nail. It is probably the most important Tsing point of them all. It is located in the depression at the junction of the anterior and middle third of the sole and in a depression between the second and third metatarso-phalangeal joints. It is the only acupoint on the sole of the foot and is of vital importance. It is said to be the foot chakra, and hence has much power that can be utilized. It is used in the general balancing of energies (superior and inferior, left and right) and in pain relief of the upper extremities. It is also an excellent point to use when calming patients if they are in a stressed state, and is extremely good in anxiety states such as claustrophobia.

Source point – Ki 3

This point is located midway between the tip of the medial malleolus and the Achilles tendon. It is a very useful point when treating acute kidney imbalance such as nephritis, low back pain and testicular discomfort. Used in stimulation it is also useful in enuresis, chronic nephritis, chronic cystitis, irregular menstruation and general weakness of the lower spine.

Tonification point – Ki 7

This point is situated on the anterior border of the Achilles tendon, 2 cun above the medial malleolus. It is a good point to use with the previous point in enuresis, night sweats, looseness of the bowel and lumbago. It is also the point that is stimulated in order to transfer energy to the liver meridian.

Great point – Ki 6

This point is situated 1 cun directly below the tip of the medial malleolus.

Uses:

1. The treatment of the sexual organs, such as painful menstruation, scrotal pain and uterine collapse.
2. Pain relief for the antero-medial aspect of the torso, pubic area and groin, genital area and adductors.
3. It is one of the key points of the eight extraordinary meridians, with its couple being Lu 7. It therefore of use, with others, in the treatment of both types of arthritis and in maintaining a healthy immune system.
4. It is one of the great 'energy' points, and as such can be used in such conditions as chronic fatigue syndrome and other conditions where lethargy and tiredness play significant roles.
5. It is a major 'focal' or visualization point when used in certain types of Tai Chi or Qi Gong.

Other important kidney points

Ki 27 is the last point on the kidney meridian. It is situated in the depression between the first rib and the lower border of the clavicle, 2 cun lateral to the midline. This point is said to be the clavicular chakra and as such is a powerful point when used locally and generally. Locally it is used in chest pain, thyroid imbalance and lower cervical stiffness. Generally it can be used, in conjunction with other points, i.e. Sp 21 and Bl 11, in the treatment of abnormalities due to an imbalance of calcium formation, e.g. Scheurmann's disease, ankylosing spondylitis and cervical spondylosis. It is said to influence the parathyroid glands and their functioning in the influence of calcium metabolism.

Pericardium meridian

The pericardium meridian is one of four non-organ channels (the others are three heater, conception and governor). It commences 1 cun lateral to the nipple and then passes into the anterior aspect of the arm and descends along the midline to the forearm and palm, terminating at the tip of the middle finger. The pericardium meridian may also be called heart constrictor or circulation/sex, and would have the abbreviations of HC or CX in these cases (Figure 3.7).

Associations

Energy type – Yin
Energy peak time – 1900 hrs
No. of points – 9
Element – Fire
Yang pairing – three heater
Sense – speech
System – circulation
Sense organ – tongue
Colour – red
Season – summer
Taste – bitter
Weather – heat
Emotional – excess joy

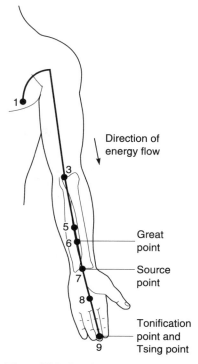

Figure 3.7 Pericardium meridian.

In practical terms, the pericardium is closely related to the heart. In Western medicine, the pericardium is seen as the protective outer covering of the heart. This is mirrored in TCM which sees the Pericardium protecting the Heart from invasion by external pathogenic factors, such as high fevers. Whereas the heart is concerned with many emotional and mental imbalances, the pericardium is basically concerned with the circulation of blood and lymph. It protects and regulates cardiac function. Because of the influence on circulation, the pericardium is chiefly concerned with the treatment of such conditions as angina, palpitation, low and high blood pressure and lymphatic congestion.

Source point – P 7

This point is situated on the transverse crease of the wrist, between the palmaris longus and flexor carpi radialis. It can be useful in the treatment of insomnia and high blood pressure.

Tonification point – P 9

This point is situated at the anterior tip of the middle finger. Its only value in acupressure is in energy balancing by passing energy through to the spleen meridian.

Great point – P 6

This point is situated 2 cun proximal to the anterior wrist crease in the midline of the forearm.

Uses:

1. Insomnia, together with Ht 7.
2. Palpitation and the pain of angina, used by itself or with LI 4.
3. Pain in the chest and costal regions.
4. Hiccups.
5. General poor circulation and breakdown of blood patency.
6. Nausea and 'travel sickness'.

It is one of the key points of the eight extra meridians being coupled with Sp 4 for treatments associated with balancing the hormonal system.

Other important pericardium points

P 3 is located in the middle of the cubital crease on the ulnar side of the biceps brachii tendon. It represents the physical aspect of the elbow chakra, being coupled with the knee chakra and the base chakra in subtle energy terms.

   P 8 is located in the middle of the palm, between the middle and ring fingers, adjacent to the third metacarpal bone. It represents the hand chakra, being coupled with the foot chakra and the crown chakra in subtle energy terms.

   The above two points are important local and distal points, their significance will be outlined in Chapter 5, describing treatment of chronic conditions.

Three heater meridian

The three heater may also be known as triple heater, triple warmer, triple energizer or by the Chinese word 'Sanjiao'. The channel commences on the ulnar border of the little finger at the nail point, it then ascends the posterior aspect of the forearm and arm, passes over the shoulder and outer border of the neck and ends at the lateral corner of the eye (Figure 3.8).

Associations

Energy type – Yang
Energy peak time – 2100 hrs
No. of points – 23
Element – Fire
Yin pairing – pericardium
Sense – speech
System – circulation
Sense organ – tongue
Colour – red
Season – summer
Taste – bitter
Weather – hot
Emotion – excess joy, euphoria

This is the second of four meridians that do not relate to an internal organ. The three heater meridian controls three areas of function. The upper heater is responsible for the intake of Chi and influences the area above the diaphragm, including the heart and lungs; the middle heater is responsible for digestive function and influences the abdomen, including the stomach,

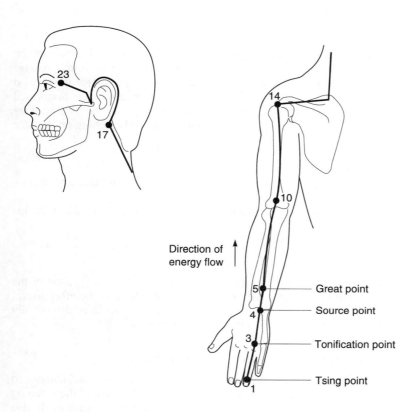

Figure 3.8 Three heater meridian.

spleen and gall bladder; the lower heater is responsible for excretion and influences the pelvic area, including the small intestine, large intestine, liver, kidneys, bladder and reproductive organs. The three heater can be likened to the manager who oversees the day-to-day workings of his or her 'team'. By ensuring that the Yang energy of the kidneys is co-ordinated appropriately, the three heater helps move Chi and maintains the ambient temperature in the body.

Source point – TH 4

This point is located in a depression of the dorsal wrist crease between extensor digitorum longus and extensor digiti minimi. It generally eliminates heat and moves Chi from one part of the heater to another. By stimulating this point it stimulates Chi in the whole of the heater. It is therefore an excellent point in the treatment of poor circulation with added cold sensations, also with the symptoms of 'hot flushes' in the menopause.

Tonification point – TH 3

This point is situated on the posterior aspect of the hand, between the fourth and fifth metacarpals and proximal to the metacarpo-phalangeal joint. It can be used as a distal point in the treatment of ear conditions and headaches. It is also one of the best points for the treatment of 'hot flushes' and general heat and redness around the head and shoulders. It is also, of course, used to pass on energy to the stomach meridian.

Great point – TH 5

This point is situated 2 cun superior to the posterior wrist crease in the midline of the forearm. It directly opposes point P 6, and a clever acupuncturist can actually lace a needle through P 6 and pierce the skin on the opposite side of the arm at TH 5. The author once saw this performed during a practical lecture at an acupuncture college, it was followed by much fainting of the viewing students and a definite blanching on the face of the recipient!

Uses:

1. As the main point for 'bringing heat down' from the face and chest – it is excellent in hot flushes.
2. Paralysis of the sternocleidomastoid and upper fibres of the trapezius muscle (torticollis).
3. Deafness due to catarrh.
4. Fever.
5. Cold hands.
6. This point (as with many great points) is one of the key points of the eight extra meridians, with GB 41 as its couple. It is therefore useful in the treatment of arthritic and hormonal conditions. It is also the key point of the crown chakra based at governor 20.

Other useful three heater meridian points

TH 17 is situated in the depression posterior to the ear lobe and anterior to the mastoid process. This is a very versatile point. It is one of the listening posts of the skull, used for the analysis of circulatory conditions. It also represents the ear chakra, being associated with the intercostal chakra at Sp 21 and also the heart chakra. Its many ranges of influence include deafness, tinnitus, facial paralysis, dry mouth and conditions associated with the upper warmer.

Gall bladder meridian

This meridian is the second longest, next to the bladder. It commences at the corner of the eye and passes to the tragus, ascends to pass around the ear and then to the occiput. It passes back over the head to the middle of the forehead, retraces its path more medially and descends to the occiput once more, passing over the shoulder into the outer aspect of the thorax, torso and abdomen. It then descends the lateral aspect of the thigh, leg and foot to end at the nail point on the lateral side of the fourth toe. the gall bladder meridian is unique in that it is the only meridian to pass down the lateral aspect of the body (Figure 3.9).

Associations

Energy type – Yang
Energy peak time – 2300 hrs
No. of points – 44
Element – Wood
Yin pairing – liver
Sense – sight

Figure 3.9 Gall bladder meridian.

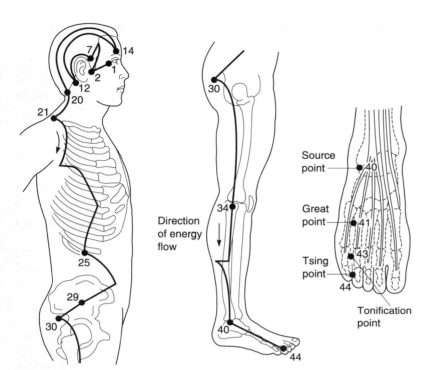

System – muscles and tendons
Sense organ – eyes
Colour – green
Season – spring
Taste – sour
Weather – wind
Emotion – anger, rage, bitterness

The gall bladder has a similar function in TCM to that of Western medicine: it stores and secretes bile that it receives from the liver and excretes it into the digestive tract to aid digestion. Excessive consumption of greasy and fatty foods can cause disharmony in the channel. The gall bladder's function is very closely allied to its Yin counterpart, the liver. Emotionally, like the liver, it is affected by constant anger, frustration, resentment and worry, giving symptoms of headache, migraine, nausea and digestive imbalance.

Source point – GB 40

This point is located anterior and inferior to the lateral malleolus, in the depression on the lateral side of the extensor digitorum longus tendon. It is indicated in acute gall bladder colic and nausea.

Tonification point – GB 43

This point is situated between the fourth and fifth metatarsal bones, 0.5 cun proximal to the margin of the web. It can be used in headaches, dizziness, chest pains and also used to pass energy onto the small intestine or three heater.

Great point – GB 41

This point is situated in the depression distal to the junction of the fourth and fifth metatarsals.

Uses:

1. In the treatment of hemi-cranial headaches, frontal headaches and shoulder pain.
2. Biliousness and colic.
3. Tinnitus (use in combination with other points).
4. Pain in the hip and along the ilio-tibial tract.
5. Conditions associated with the emotions of anger, rage, frustration and worry.
6. It is the key point of one of the eight extra meridians, coupled with TH 5, and as such is used in the treatment of certain types of arthritis and hormonal imbalance.

Other important gall bladder points

GB 2 is located in a depression when the mouth is opened just behind the mandible condyle. It is a very good local point for certain types of deafness, tinnitus, otitis media and used in TMJ (temporo-mandibular joint) imbalance.

GB 7 is located at the crossing of the horizontal line of the auricle and the line that projects from the anterior auricle. This point has already been mentioned as one of the listening post points, used in muscle and tendon energy analysis.

GB 14 is located 1 cun above the mid-point of the eyebrow. This point is very useful in the treatment of stress-related conditions and in relaxation techniques. It will be fully discussed in Chapter 6.

GB 20 is situated between the origins of the sternocleidomastoid and trapezius muscles on the occiput. It is an excellent point for the relief of neck tension, cervical pain and torticollis as well as the main point for occipital headaches.

GB 21 is located midway between the seventh cervical spinous process and the acromium process at the highest point of the shoulder. This is a common trigger point in the treatment of neck tension, muscular spasm and neck pain. Deep pressure on this point helps to energize the arm and hands when they are cold.

Other influential points on this meridian are **GB 29**, **GB 30** and **GB 34**. Their chief actions lie in the treatment of hip and knee joint pain and several tendinous conditions. They are discussed fully in the previous book.

Liver meridian

The liver meridian commences at the nail point on the lateral aspect of the great toe, passes along the medial side of the foot, leg and thigh to the external genitalia. It then ascends the abdomen to end at the sixth intercostal space on the lateral chest wall (Figure 3.10).

Figure 3.10 Liver meridian.

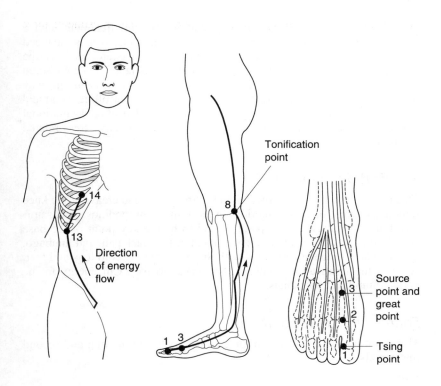

Associations

Energy type – Yin
Energy peak time – 0100 hrs
No. of points – 14
Element – Wood
Yang pairing – gall bladder
Sense – sight
System – muscles and tendons
Colour – green
Season – spring
Taste – sour
Weather – wind
Emotion – anger, bitterness, sadness, frustration

The liver is probably the most complicated organ, next to the brain, in the body. Memories flood back of trying to learn the main 24 functions of the liver by making up a very rude mnemonic. It has many more functions than 24, but they are the main ones. A major function of the liver is to regulate the amount of blood in circulation. This varies, obviously, with activity of the muscles. The liver, therefore, stores and releases blood at will. In women, because of this role in storing and releasing blood, the liver is closely associated with menstruation and many gynaecological conditions occur due to liver Chi imbalance. The emotions are very important when it comes to liver meridian imbalance. People who worry, get angry, have long-term frustrations and bitterness, tend to have stagnation of liver Chi. This gives rise to heavy eyes, headaches, migraines, weak musculature and lethargy. If these emotional traits are combined with a faulty eating pattern, the liver can become very sick. Always with acupressure treatment, advice as to a well-balanced diet must take priority. When the liver is balanced and functioning well, then effective control can be exercised over the events in our life and response to sudden changes are taken in a considered and flexible manner. On the other hand, if liver function is in any way impaired, there can be a tendency to becoming over-controlling, rigid and inflexible. This may lead to outbursts of anger and irrational emotional reactions. Liver disharmonies are always present in any stress-related disorder.

Tonification point – Li 8

This point is situated at the medial end of the transverse crease of the knee joint in a depression at the anterior border of the semi-tendinosis and semi-membranosis muscles. This point is said to be the key point of the base chakra. It is used clinically in the treatment of low back pain and lumbago. It is also useful, when combined with St 36, in treating cold legs and feet. As it is the tonification point, it also serves to pass Chi energy to the pericardium/heart meridians.

Source and great point – Li 3

This point is situated at the proximal aspect between the first and second metatarsals.

Uses:

1. Calming the nerves and easing restlessness and anxiety, either by itself or in combination with LI 4.
2. Headaches, especially behind the eyes and those due to a hangover. It is interesting to note that one of the best homoeopathic remedies for a hangover is nux vomica. This is said to be a 'liver' remedy in that it is useful for headaches and also ill temper. I have often indicated to my students that nux vomica is to be thought of if the symptoms indicate the use of Li 3. This is often a very good combination of points when commencing a treatment on someone who is anxious, frightened or stressed.
3. Mastitis.
4. Muscular tiredness and 'all gone' sensation.
5. Cramp – this is *the* specific point for cramp regardless of where it is in the body, but it is particularly effective in the treatment of calf cramp. Many a sleepless night has been saved with the knowledge of this point. Very gentle touch is required for up to 3 minutes, with *no* stimulation.
6. Either by itself or in combination with other points in menopausal and menstruation abnormalities.

Li 3 is one of *the* very great points in acupressure because it can be used to good effect in many conditions. It is particularly effective when used in tandem with LI 4.

Other important liver points

Li 2 is located 0.5 cun proximal to the margin of the web between the first and second toes. It is useful to treat Yang conditions associated with liver imbalance, namely redness and swelling of the eye, intercostal pain, urethritis and insomnia.

Li 13 is located at the end of the 11th rib. This can be a very tender point. It is the 'alarm' point for the spleen and is therefore useful in the treatment of blood disorders and lethargy.

Lung meridian

The lung meridian commences on the lateral aspect of the chest 2 cun lateral to the nipple line and descends the arm on its antero-lateral aspect, passing over the thenar eminence to end at the nail point on the lateral aspect of the thumb (Figure 3.11).

Associations

Energy type – Yin
Energy peak time – 0300
No. of points – 11
Element – Metal
Yang pairing – large intestine
Sense – smell
System – skin
Sense organ – nose
Colour – white
Season – autumn (fall)
Taste – pungent
Weather – dryness
Emotion – grief, sadness, shame

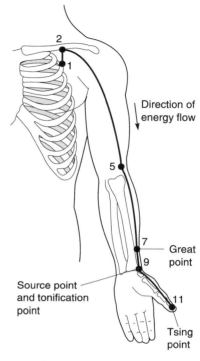

Figure 3.11 Lung meridian.

The lung channel is recognized as having similar properties in TCM and orthodox medicine, with a few differences. The lungs govern the inhalation of pure Chi from the air and the exhalation of impure Chi. The main difference in TCM is that it is the Chi that is obtained from the air that is important, not just the oxygen. Secondly, the spleen sends up the Chi extracted from food to the lungs, where it combines with the pure Chi inhaled in the air to be spread to all parts of the body. If there is an imbalance of Chi in the lungs, this can lead to general symptoms of Chi deficiency affecting the whole body causing tiredness and lethargy as well as the characteristic symptoms associated with lung conditions such as mucous, shortness of breath and bronchitis. Lung energy deals with the nose, nasal passages, sinuses, throat and bronchus as well as the lungs. Lung energy also deals with the skin – after all the skin is said to be the third lung and one of the main organs of excretion. In combination with the large intestine, the lung meridian is dedicated to excretion of impure Chi.

Source point and tonification point – Lu 9

This point is situated in the depression on the radial side of the radial artery on the anterior wrist crease. This very useful point is indicated in stimulating energy to the lungs and is useful to help the symptoms of chronic bronchitis. It is also used to pass energy on to the kidney meridian.

Great point – Lu 7

This point is located on the radial side of the forearm, 1.5 cun proximal to the transverse wrist crease.

Uses:

1.   In the treatment of obstructive airways diseases such as acute and chronic bronchitis, emphysema and asthma. Lu 7 is said to be the 'oxygen' point of the lung and is therefore useful in such cases.
2.   Congestive sinusitis and catarrh.
3.   Useful as an emergency point (with LI 4 and Lu 1) in the easing of acute asthma symptoms.
4.   It is the key point of the conception meridian with its couple being Ki 6. It is therefore helpful in many chest conditions and chronic hormonal imbalances.
5.   Headaches of the 'brain fog' type – used either by itself or in conjunction with LI 4.
6.   Useful in facial pain, toothache and shoulder pain.

Other important lung points

Lu 1 is situated 2 cun lateral to the nipple line in the second intercostal space. It is known as the master point of the lungs, as it can be used to tonify the breathing mechanism. It should be tonified in chronic bronchitis, breathlessness, panting and exhaustion and sedated in acute symptoms of tightness of the chest with much muscle spasm.

Large intestine meridian

The large intestine (large bowel or colon) meridian commences on the lateral nail point of the index finger, passes between the first and second metacarpals into the postero-lateral aspect of the forearm and arm, crosses the shoulder joint from posterior to anterior and ascends the lateral side of the neck, crossing to the opposite side to end just lateral to the nasal ala. It is unique in meridians in that it is the only one that crosses the midline. Therefore the last point, LI 20 regulates the flow of lung energy on the opposite side of the body (Figure 3.12).

Associations

Energy type – Yang
Energy peak time – 0500 hrs
No. of points – 20
Element – Metal
Yin pairing – lung
Sense – smell
System – skin
Sense organ – nose
Colour – white
Season – autumn (fall)
Taste – pungent
Weather – dryness
Emotion – grief, sadness

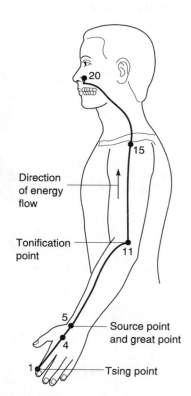

Direction of energy flow

Tonification point

Source point and great point

Tsing point

Figure 3.12 Large intestine meridian.

The large intestine receives the impure Chi from the small intestine and further refines it to extract further pure fluids or essence, it then secretes the impure as faeces. It is the most important meridian that deals with excretion, not just physical waste but also of emotions. It therefore deals with conditions of the large bowel, lungs, skin, sinuses, air passages and the varying emotions that come with being unable to excrete and 'get rid of' waste (impure) thoughts. These include depression, anxiety and sadness. The traditional TCM 'mental' association is grief. It can be seen, therefore, that many bowel and skin abnormalities come because of emotional causes and not necessarily because of faulty eating.

Tsing point – LI 1

This point is situated on the radial side of the index finger. It is used specifically in toothache and pain around the mouth, and is also a revival point in unconsciousness.

Tonification point – LI 11

This point is located at the lateral edge of the elbow crease when the elbow is flexed. It is used as a general 'calming' point either by itself or with LI 4. It is also used to pass energy on to the bladder meridian.

Source point and great point – LI 4

This point is situated at the highest point on the mound of the first interosseus muscle with the thumb and forefinger opposed.

Uses:

1. Pain relief for the face, head, front and lateral aspect of the shoulder and elbow.
2. Pain relief for the dorsum of the neck and occiput, also sinusitis and toothache of the lower jaw.
3. Constipation and large bowel conditions.
4. Skin conditions, especially acne of the face.
5. Localized tendinitis.
6. It is also used in combination with other points as follows: with Li 3 in calming, with Lu 7 in easing throat congestion and pain, with Si 2 or Si 3 in nosebleeds, with Ht 7 in insomnia or nightmares, with Sp 6 in many gynaecological conditions.

This point is affectionately called 'the great eliminator', and is probably the most used point in acupuncture and acupressure simply because of its power and versatility. It is, however, contraindicated in pregnancy (except at time of childbirth) and during menstruation.

Other important large intestine points

LI 15 is situated at the antero-inferior border of the acromio-clavicular joint, inferior to the acromion process when the arm is in adduction. It is a very powerful point and can be used for painful conditions around the neck (anterior and posterior), throat and head, as well as being used as a local point in shoulder pain. It is also one of the minor chakra points (shoulder chakra). It is associated with the throat chakra and deals with elimination, easing tension and anxiety and in skin and bowel conditions.

LI 20 is located between the naso-labial groove and the midpoint of the outer border of the nasal ala. It is particularly effective when used as a local point in rhinitis, blocked nose and toothache. It can also be used in allergic conditions in combination with LI 4 and LI 11.

The extra meridians

It has already been pointed out that as well as the 12 bilateral 'organ' meridians, there are another eight that are not related to an individual organ. Six of the eight are bilateral and are made up of composite points from the 12 organ meridians. Although they are very useful in acupuncture, their role in acupressure is very limited, so they are not mentioned, as it would only serve to confuse the embattled reader still further. The two extra meridians that need to be discussed are the two unilateral channels called governor and conception.

Governor meridian

The governor meridian commences between the tip of the coccyx and the anus, proceeds up the midline of the spinal column, passing over the head to end at Gov 28 which lies between the upper lip and the gum. The governor channel may also be called governing, du mai or back midline. Its abbreviations can be Du, GV or Gov. So as not to confuse GV with CV, for this series of books, the abbreviation of Gov is used (Figure 3.13).

Figure 3.13 Governor meridian.

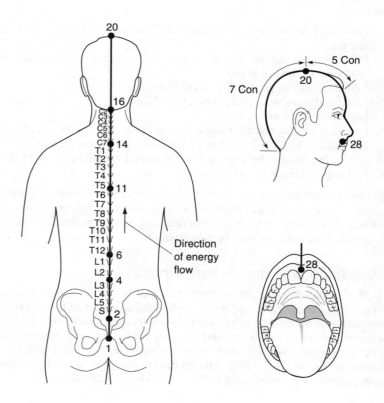

Associations

Energy type – Yang
No. of points – 28
Yin pairing – conception
Key point – Si 3
Extra key point – Bl 62

There are no source and great points as such, because there isn't an affinity to a particular organ.

Important governor meridian points

Gov 2 is situated at the junction between the sacrum and the coccyx. This represents an extremely important point. It is said to be the physical counterpart of the base (muladhara) chakra and is significant in the treatment of all spinal conditions. In general medical conditions, it is of immense importance in the creation of energy, not only to the spine but to the rest of the body. It could be considered in virtually all chronic diseases. The downside in using this point more often is its anatomical positioning. If the practitioner is at all perturbed about using it, the two golden rules are (a) make sure that the patient is fully aware that you are going to use this point before it is stimulated – never ever touch the point without their prior knowledge or agreement, (b) it is also advisable to have a chaperone either in the room with you or nearby.

Gov 4 is located between the spinous processes of L2 and L3. This point has an affinity with kidney energy and is closely associated with Bl 23, which lies at the same level of the spine. It is used to help with lethargy and tiredness, also 'adrenal burnout' (see Chapter 6), stimulation required here. When used in sedation, it can be used in calming and as a stress release point.

Gov 11 is situated below the spinous process of the fifth thoracic vertebra. This point is directly linked to heart energy and can be used in stimulating massage in fainting, swooning and sudden cerebral anaemia. It raises arterial tension by causing the production of adrenalin, so it is very good in the treatment of chronic anxiety. It is one of the master points in certain forms of martial arts.

Gov 14 is located between the spinous processes of C7 and T1. It is said to be the reunion point of all the Yang meridians and is a most influential energy point. It is the posterior aspect of the throat chakra and has a direct energy link with the thyroid gland. When stimulated it can provide 'instant' short-term energy. When sedated, it is one of the very great points used in stress release.

Gov 16 is located directly below the occipital protuberance, in the midline. It may be used as a local point in the treatment of headaches and cervical spine stiffness. Its use as a general point is where it is such a wonderful point. It is considered to be one of the great points in the treatment of neurological imbalance as well as stress-related conditions. Full details of using this point are discussed in Chapter 6.

Gov 20 is situated 5 cun behind the anterior hairline and 7 cun above the posterior hairline. This is a *huge* point in acupressure, and healing in general. It represents the crown (sahasrara) chakra in esoteric medicine which deals with the spirituality of a person. In TCM terms, it is said to be the reunion point for all yang meridians. When stimulated, it draws energy to the head from the base of the spine, being very good in the treatment of

Figure 3.14 Key points.

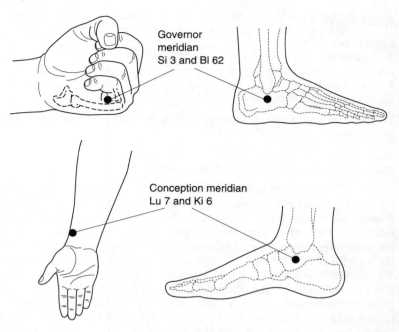

haemorrhoids and low back pain. When sedated, it eases headaches and fullness in the head. It is most commonly used in stress conditions.

The so-called key point (or opening point) for the governor channel is Si 3. There is also a secondary key point of Bl 62 (see Figure 3.14). In order to have more effect in using the governor channel and to create more energy there in the first place, these two points must be stimulated for up to half a minute before any of the governor points are used. Experience has shown that this procedure seems to be very effective.

Conception meridian

The conception meridian commences at the centre of the perineum, between the anus and the scrotum. It passes up the anterior midline of the body to the neck and lower jaw to the outside of the lower lip. It is sometimes called the ren mai, directing or central channel. The abbreviations used can be CV, Ren or Con. The abbreviation of Con is used as CV is often confused with GV (Figure 3.15).

Associations

Energy type – Yin
No. of points – 24
Yang pairing – governor
Key point – Lu 7
Extra key point – Ki 6

Important conception meridian points

Virtually every conception point can be said to have some importance in acupressure due to the energy affinity of the underlying organs, but some

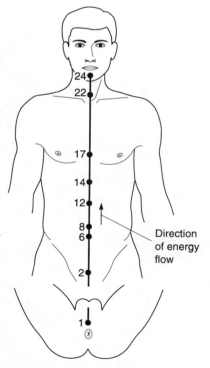

Figure 3.15 Conception meridian.

points are more effective than others when dealing with touch therapies. This is sometimes in contradiction to the major points that are useful in acupuncture.

Con 2 is situated on the upper border of the symphysis pubis. This represents another *huge* point in acupressure. Like many of the important conception points, it is the physical counterpart of the base (muladhara) chakra and as such is very useful in dealing with most chronic disease. Stimulating massage should be performed in all chronic conditions, especially those involving hereditary, kidney, bladder, spinal and neurological conditions. It is useful to commence a treatment by stimulating this point. As was pointed out with Gov 2, the downside of this point is its anatomical position. The same advice for treatment holds good for this point. Always inform the patient what your intentions are before you touch them. A lawsuit is not something that should be sought. The ways of using this point, and others, are outlined in Chapter 4.

Con 6 is situated 1.5 cun below the umbilicus. It is a very important energy point, being the anterior sacral chakra. It is also known as the *hara* point or the Sea of Energy. It is used with sedative massage in general relaxation and insomnia and with stimulating massage in order to bring energy to the areas below the point. This can be very useful in chronic pelvic disorders, chronic bladder conditions, as well as lower spinal stiffness and coldness. A magic point!

Con 14 is located 6 cun superior to the umbilicus or just below the xiphoid process (in people who possess it). This point is said to be directly linked with the solar plexus (coeliac plexus) and as such is a very powerful energy point. It can be sedated in agitation, anxiety and acute stomach pain, and stimulated to provide energy to the stomach, liver and pancreas. It is the first aid point for people who experience a sudden hypoglycaemic experience. Care should be taken when using this point. Never stimulate when the patient is agitated or confused.

Con 17 is located on the sternum at the level with the nipples at the level of the fourth intercostal space. It is associated with the heart (anahata) chakra and is a useful point in stress-related illness. It is also concerned with circulatory disorders and is particularly useful in sedation in acute asthmatic attacks.

Con 22 is situated at the centre of the suprasternal fossa 0.5 cun above the sternal notch. This point is the anterior throat (visshuda) chakra and is directly linked with the thyroid gland. It can be used in both stimulation and sedation in balancing the energy in this endocrine gland. It is an excellent energy point and can be used with patients who suffer from desperate lethargy, 'tired all the time' syndrome and obesity due to glandular imbalance. It is also very useful in the treatment of throat and upper bronchial conditions.

Reflexes

In the previous two chapters, the concept of reflexes as being reflected pathways and points was discussed. It has already been pointed out that reflexes represent wonderful points that can be used in acupressure healing, being equal in importance to meridian acupoints. Chapter 1 dealt with using the foot and hand reflexes as areas of analysis and diagnosis and it is not intended to discuss these well known reflexes any further. Therapists who wish to know more about the rudiments of foot and hand reflexology can easily purchase one of scores of books on the market that deal with this. In the later chapter dealing with the treatment of individual conditions, the foot and hand reflexes will be mentioned. This chapter, however, deals with using some of the lesser known reflexes on the hands, skull, face, ear and body in general. Some of them can be used in analysis and all of them can be used in treatment.

Face and skull reflexes

Several interpretations of facial and skull reflex points exist, each depicting a different philosophy. These different approaches may be based on traditional Chinese, Japanese, Ayurvedic and Shaman medicine that have been handed down from generation to generation. There are also some more modern concepts that are based on several therapists' interpretations. The following two approaches represent composites of many different philosophies. The author has been using these clinically and in teaching for several years but has not had the opportunity to submit them to print.

Figure 3.16 shows single point and area reflexes of the skull and face. They are used strictly in the treatment of acute or 'here and now' conditions. They are not supposed to be used in chronic ongoing conditions, but personal research does not dismiss this idea. The reflexes do not relate to individual organs or energy channels as such, but deal with acute conditions. Many of the points are the same as meridian acupoints – both meridian and non-meridian, some have been based on an old shamanic chart, others are based on applied kinesiology and yet others based on the 'trial and error' philosophy. Point no. 2 for instance is

Figure 3.16 Face and head reflexes.

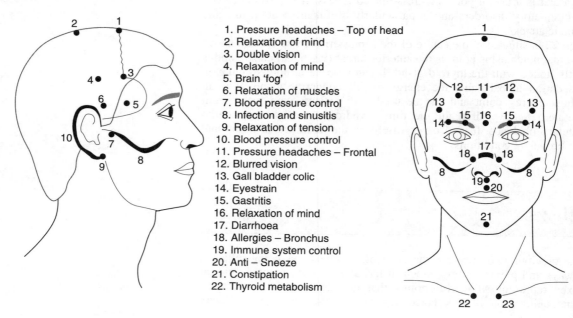

1. Pressure headaches – Top of head
2. Relaxation of mind
3. Double vision
4. Relaxation of mind
5. Brain 'fog'
6. Relaxation of muscles
7. Blood pressure control
8. Infection and sinusitis
9. Relaxation of tension
10. Blood pressure control
11. Pressure headaches – Frontal
12. Blurred vision
13. Gall bladder colic
14. Eyestrain
15. Gastritis
16. Relaxation of mind
17. Diarrhoea
18. Allergies – Bronchus
19. Immune system control
20. Anti – Sneeze
21. Constipation
22. Thyroid metabolism

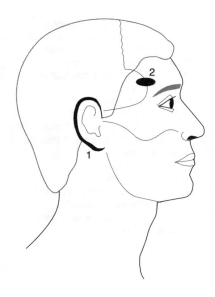

1. Blood circulation
2. Sciatica
3. Reproductive organs
4. Memory
5. Autonomic nervous system
6. Pelvic region
7. Insomnia
8. Headaches
9. Stomach
10. Large intestine
11. Kidney
12. Large and small intestines
13. Stomach
14. Spleen
15. Pancreas
16. Lungs
17. Heart
18. Liver and gall bladder
19. Lymphatics
20. Bladder
21. Large intestine
22. Sexual
23. Thyroid

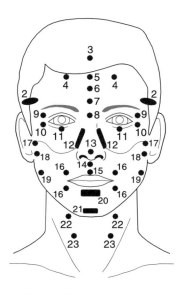

Figure 3.17 Face reflexes.

governor 20, point no. 16 is Extra 1 (brow chakra) and point 13 is Gall Bladder 14. As with all acute and painful conditions, the reflected points and areas need to be sedated. This means that the points need to be touched very gently for about 5–10 minutes. A 'change of emphasis' should occur under the fingers after about 3–4 minutes. Experience shows that reflex points are not so quick as acupoints when it comes to the change of emphasis and subsequent brain wave alteration. These points should be used in conjunction with others.

Figure 3.17 looks more like someone with chickenpox than a chart of facial reflexes. These reflexes are based on traditional Chinese and Japanese charts and are used for analysis and treatment of chronic and 'ongoing' conditions. Experience has shown that they are not too useful in the treatment of acute conditions. In analytical mode, if the point exhibits tenderness to gentle palpation, it should then be treated with stimulating massage for up to 2 minutes. It is recommended that patients are taught these 'trigger' points so that they can be encouraged to self-treat whilst at home, away from the therapist's clutches! It is advisable for them to stimulate each point for up to 2 minutes every 2 hours. The patient will experience a warm glow in the area of massage and sometimes in the area that is being affected at a distance.

Hand reflexes

The reflex areas of the hand were discussed in a previous chapter. This chapter deals with reflected points of the hand that are based on traditional Chinese and Japanese charts (see Figure 3.18). These points may be used for both analysis and treatment and are best used in the treatment of acute conditions. Like other reflected areas of the body, with a few exceptions, the periphery of the body is represented on the dorsum of the hand and the internal organs are represented on the palmar aspect. There are some

Figure 3.18 Hand reflexes.

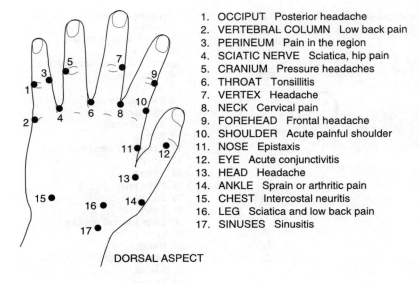

1. OCCIPUT   Posterior headache
2. VERTEBRAL COLUMN   Low back pain
3. PERINEUM   Pain in the region
4. SCIATIC NERVE   Sciatica, hip pain
5. CRANIUM   Pressure headaches
6. THROAT   Tonsillitis
7. VERTEX   Headache
8. NECK   Cervical pain
9. FOREHEAD   Frontal headache
10. SHOULDER   Acute painful shoulder
11. NOSE   Epistaxis
12. EYE   Acute conjunctivitis
13. HEAD   Headache
14. ANKLE   Sprain or arthritic pain
15. CHEST   Intercostal neuritis
16. LEG   Sciatica and low back pain
17. SINUSES   Sinusitis

DORSAL ASPECT

18. CHEST   Acute asthma
19. G.I. TRACT   Abdominal pain
20. LARGE INTESTINE   Pain
21. SMALL INTESTINE   Diarrhoea
22. HEART   Palpitation
23. LYMPHATIC DISORDERS
24. SPLEEN   Blood disease
25. LIVER   Jaundice
26. KIDNEY   Pain
27. BLADDER   Cystitis
28. LUNG   Chronic coughing
29. THROAT   Sore, bronchitis
30. MOUTH   Toothache
31. PALPITATION   Dizziness
32. HYSTERIA   Emotional disturbance
33. EXCESSIVE SWEATING
34. COMMON COLD   Rhinitis
35. STOMACH   Pain, vomiting
36. HEEL   Sprained ankle

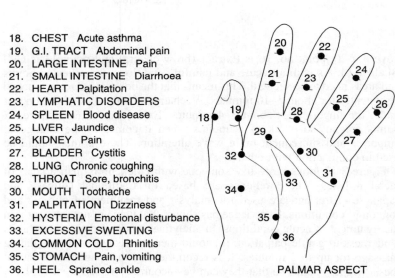

PALMAR ASPECT

meridian acupoints represented as reflex points, e.g. point 2 is Si 3, point 13 is LI 4 and point 15 is TH 3. Some of the other points are called 'extra' points in TCM. In analysis mode, the points should be pressed and gently massaged for just a couple of seconds in order to evoke a response or not. If the response is positive (thus showing that the associated body part needs treatment and energy balancing), the reflex should be acutely tender. If there is no or little response, this shows that treatment is not required. When using the reflexes in treatment mode, the points should be gently pressed and rubbed (or just held) for anything up to 5 minutes. The associated organ or body part should feel much more relaxed when using this method. This particular aspect of treatment serves as a very good overture in a whole treatment plan prior to treating the cause of the imbalance. As has been stated many times before, it is pointless treating the cause of the condition without giving the patient some kind of relief. The two *can* go hand in hand.

Ear reflexes

The art of using the ear for treatment with touch therapy is part of TCM. The ear can be used as a reflected area for both diagnosis and treatment. As with all the reflected areas and pathways on the body, the whole of the body can be mapped within the ear, with the protected organs being at the centre and the peripheral organs being in the outside. The ear reflexes are said to represent an inverted foetus (see Figure 3.19), with the head being in the lobe, the internal organs being 'protected' within the concha and the limbs and spine being around the scaphoid fossa. It is important that before the therapist proceeds headlong into treatment, the ear is looked at and tentatively felt. Be on the look-out for areas of redness, puffiness or skin abrasions – these all mean something. Redness indicates that the associated organs/areas are acutely inflamed; puffiness means that there is a chronic condition; and skin abrasion can mean a serious condition with the associated organ. Skin abrasions could also mean the person has eczema – common sense is needed here! Once the reflected point is found, the therapist may use either the pad of the little finger or a cotton bud to exert a little pressure on the point in order to effect pain relief in the affected part. This technique may last a few minutes. It may be wise to introduce some gentle movement to initiate the healing response, but once the patient's discomfort starts to ease, the finger or cotton bud should be kept perfectly still.

Chapman's reflexes

These important reflexes were discussed in the previous book because of their importance in the treatment of musculo-skeletal conditions. The author has also used these reflexes successfully for several years in the treatment of medical conditions with acupressure and reflextherapy, and so they are mentioned again.

Dr Frank Chapman, an osteopath, discovered the 'Chapman's reflexes' in the 1930s. He found that by stimulating a specific point, it would increase lymphatic drainage in a specific organ. The locations of these reflexes are primarily along the anterior intercostal spaces down to the pubis, and posteriorly down the spine adjacent to the spinous processes and over the transverse processes. There are some other reflexes located down the legs, down the sternum and underneath the clavicle (see Figure 3.20). Active reflexes can usually be palpated and are quite tender, especially those on the anterior surface. The tenderness is usually in direct ratio to the chronicity and severity of the condition. The reflexes on the anterior of the body are small and located in the subcutaneous fat, and often feel like a small pea or bean. The posterior ones are usually less tender and more difficult to palpate – the feeling here is more diffuse and less specific. Many of the reflected points and areas are linked with more than one organ/system/meridian. Modern applied kinesiology has called these reflexes 'neuro-lymphatic reflexes', as it was shown that each reflex was associated with both an internal organ and muscle group via the autonomic nervous system. Treatment of Chapman's reflexes is done with the finger

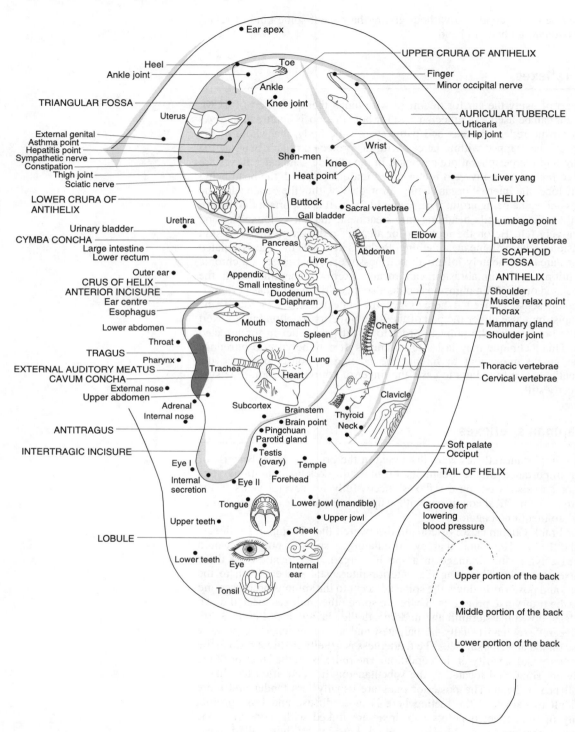

Figure 3.19 Ear reflexes.

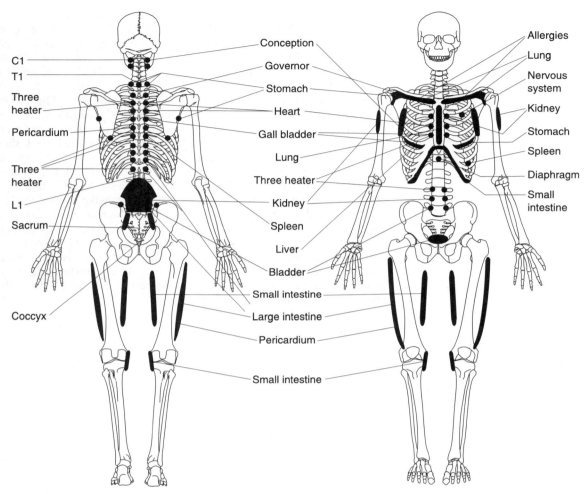

Figure 3.20 Chapmans (neuro-lymphatic) reflexes.

pads in a rotatory manner. The reflex will need a very firm pressure, especially in chronic conditions – it is hardly a subtle treatment, and is, in fact, one of the most painful procedures that can be performed in the whole field of 'bodywork'. The good news, though, is that it works!

There are two ways in which Chapman's reflexes may be used – either by massaging the points directly associated with the organ/system to improve the lymphatic congestion in a specific region or by giving a full body massage. The latter is far more beneficial in general terms. Although some points are quite painful, the whole procedure should, with practice, take no more than a couple of minutes. It is a wonderful way to improve lymphatic circulation in the patient who has a chronic disability. They tend to feel better instantly. They must be warned, however, that it is a painful procedure. The areas that are most painful are those associated with the pericardium and large intestine on the outside and inside regions of the legs, and the areas under the clavicle that are associated with the lungs, stomach, governor meridian and also with allergies.

When treating specific areas, each area associated with a system/meridian/organ should be massaged in turn for up to half a minute per area before proceeding to the next one. Strictly speaking, the areas associated with the conception, governor, nervous system, three heater and 'allergies' do not relieve lymphatic congestion within that system. Experience has shown that when these areas are massaged, it gives a beneficial effect to the muscles that are associated with that particular meridian. The 'nervous system' point over the left aspect of the chest is used mostly in stress-related conditions. The 'allergies' area underneath the clavicle and medial aspect of the shoulder is shared with stomach, governor and lung. It should be used in any congestive condition associated with the lungs, e.g. bronchitis or any allergic condition, be it food related or not. This area is extremely tender in such patients and care should be taken not to press too hard in the first part of the session. The client may make a quick exit! Like most of the other reflected areas, the patient can be encouraged to massage these points at home. Their pressure will not be so strong as the therapist's, unless they are masochists! Chapman's reflexes can be used to great advantage in the treatment of dis-ease. As well as being clinically advantageous, the techniques used will satisfy the client who has a 'no pain – no gain' attitude to treatment. It is the perfect foil for all the 'subtle' energy acupressure that is performed.

4

Treatment of acute conditions

Acute medical conditions represent any syndrome that has an overall Yang influence. For a condition to be termed 'acute' there has to be pain, discomfort and temporary alteration of lifestyle. The patient/client may suffer the acute symptoms on a periodic basis or it could be a 'one-off' situation. The symptoms are not so deep and long-standing as to warrant it becoming a chronic condition. A good way of defining an acute syndrome is to call it a 'here and now' situation that needs to be addressed in the first instance. Virtually every chronic condition has acute symptomatic overtones, but the treatment of chronic conditions with acupressure and reflextherapy is quite different from the treatment of acute ones. A golden rule of practice is to treat the acute symptoms first – firstly because they are much easier to treat, secondly because they are often the presenting symptoms of a condition and are the ones that the patient *demands* to be addressed initially, and thirdly because the acute symptoms of any condition represent the ones that the body is attempting to express and *must* be corrected. In saying this, it is vital that the therapist appreciates that the acute symptoms *do not* necessarily represent the condition itself; they should never be suppressed but should be eased by using the patient's own Chi energy.

Assessment of acute conditions

Before the acute condition can be successfully treated, the therapist should spend a couple of minutes in assessing the situation. There is nothing worse than to get 'stuck in' with the patient before the rationale of treatment is known thoroughly. The assessment is based on the principles of (a) look, (b) listen and (c) palpate. The 'look' and 'listen' will be discussed in the treatment of chronic conditions in the next chapter. Palpation should consist of the following:

1. Tsing points.
2. Abdominal alarm points.

3. Reflex points of the foot, hand, face/skull.
4. Listening post points.

It is not essential to cover all the above, but positive feedback on them should show where the cause of the acute discomfort is. Each of the points should show exquisite tenderness in the positive reactions. When this occurs, the related or associated organ/meridian should be treated.

Principles of treatment

The principles of treatment in acute conditions are:

(a) To balance the energy in the organ/system involved. This is usually by reducing the excess Yang energy.
(b) To support the energetic supply of the associated organ/system in order that symptoms do not re-appear.
(c) To balance the energy of the body in general.

This can be achieved by doing the following in the order as shown:

1. Meridian massage of the associated channels.
2. Local and distal acupressure.
3. Massaging special acupoints or reflex points for the specific condition.
4. Giving stimulating massage to the source or great point.
5. General energy balancing using the Sheng cycle of the five elements (Yang meridians).

1. Meridian massage

Once the aims of the treatment have been established and it is known which organ(s) is/are to be treated, e.g. stomach energy in gastritis, uterus energy in period pain, bladder energy in cystitis etc., the associated meridian(s) are massaged. This can be done with a broad hand sweep down the meridian *against* the flow of energy. As it does not have to be totally accurate, it is not necessary to perform it with the finger pads or to press with any degree of pressure. If necessary, it can be done through clothing – experience has shown that it is just as effective. Three or four sweeps of the bilateral or unilateral channels are sufficient. The meridians chosen are the ones that supply the affected organ plus any others that can be beneficial.

2. Local and distal acupressure

Sedation is the key in the successful treatment of acute conditions. The best way to achieve this is by local and distal acupressure. Place the middle finger of one hand on an acupoint close to the painful or inflamed area and the middle finger of the other hand on the best distal point. This could be a point on the same vertical zone, same meridian, a great point, nearest chakra point, or a foot, hand or facial reflex. Each condition is different and only experience will tell which one is best for a particular condition. In the examples of acute conditions later in the chapter the points that are indicated are those which I have found with experience seem to be the best and most effective. It may be necessary to perform some gentle rotatory or stimulating massage on the distal point for about 20 seconds or so before settling down to balance between the two points. An energy balance is achieved when the sensation under one finger pad matches the sensation under the other one. This could take up to 3–4 minutes to achieve so do not be in a hurry to complete the task or to *will* it on. As mentioned in a previous chapter, there will often be a 'change of emphasis' taking place; this is a very good sign and is often a signal that the excess Yang within the organ/area has been harmonized. The patient should now be feeling a little easier.

3. Specific acupoints massage

These are points that historically have an influence on the condition. They should be massaged quite gently for a couple of minutes, or until the patient informs you that the pain has eased.

4. Great point or source point massage

The great or source point (whichever is the better) of the corresponding meridian of the organ or the area that is being treated is now stimulated. This can be achieved by using either finger pad or thumb pad massage on the appropriate point for about half a minute. The therapist and patient will know when the desired effect has been achieved when the patient indicates a warm glow feeling coupled with relaxation.

5. General energy balancing

A very useful conclusion in the treatment of any acute medical condition is the energy balance of the whole body by using the Yang meridians on the 'Sheng' cycle of the law of five elements. Figure 1.4 on page 13 shows this law in diagrammatic form. In order to energy balance around the Sheng (engendering) cycle, the middle finger pads are placed on any two adjacent tonification points in the circle, e.g. LI 11 and Bl 67, and held for about 20 seconds. There is no need to hold any longer than this and there does not have to be any change of energy emphasis. After about 20 seconds, take the hand away from LI 11 and place it on the next point in the cycle – GB 43. Repeat this procedure until the five-element cycle is completed. When it comes to using the points on the Fire element, there is a choice of using either the three heater (TH 3) or the small intestine (Si 3) – use either *but not both*. It should take no more than a couple of minutes to complete it, but it is extremely rewarding for the patient. They can also be instructed to do it as a home exercise – try to demonstrate it without getting into knots! (See Figure 4.1.)

Treatment of acute medical conditions

Below are a number of acute conditions that the therapist is likely to be asked to treat on a regular basis, either as an individual condition or part of the more complex chronic condition scenario. Although this book is

Figure 4.1 Tonification points.

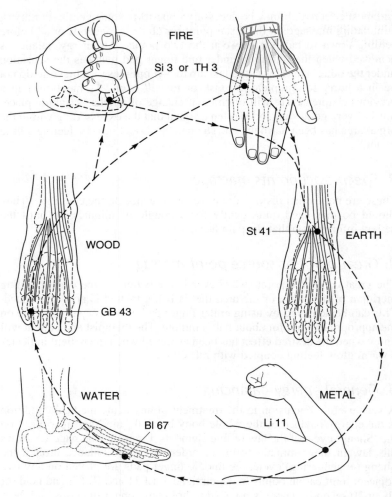

dedicated to the medical professional, certain conditions are included that would not necessarily be met in the treatment room. Advice on the treatment of, say, the common cold is given purely as a useful self-help procedure for both therapist and patient. The points used in this section (and the next chapter) represent the ones that the author uses in these conditions. They are derived from personal experience as being *the* ones that do the trick.

Respiratory conditions

Acute asthma

An acute asthmatic attack can be one of the most awful of life experiences. This section deals just with the treatment of the acute episode and is not concerned with the causes – be they allergic, psychosomatic or hereditary. The treatment of chronic asthma will be given in the next chapter. (See Figure 4.2.)

The treatment for acute asthma is as follows:

1. The associated meridian is the *lung* meridian. This should be massaged or stroked three or four times from the thumb towards the front of the chest.
2. There is an exception to the rule straightaway here. Instead of using the local and distal points next, it is essential that the anxiety of the situation is dealt with immediately. This is best done by holding both Ki 1 points on the soles of the feet. After a couple of minutes of gentle massage and holding, the patient should be feeling quite a bit easier.
3. The local point is Lu 1 and the best distal point is LI 4. Hold these two points for a couple of minutes or until a change of emphasis is felt. Do

Figure 4.2 Points used in acute asthma.

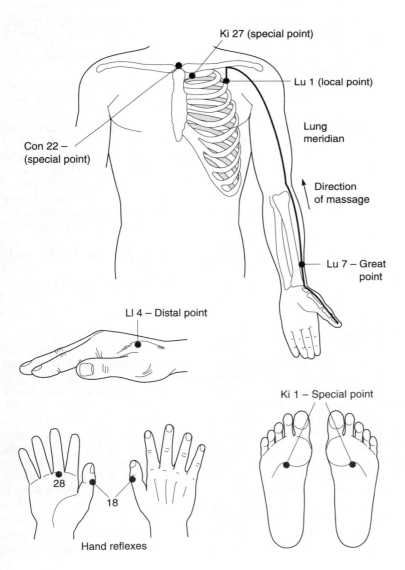

not use LI 4 if the patient is pregnant or in the early stages of a period. Use LI 11 (at the outer bend of the elbow) as an alternative.

4. The first two now need to be supported by using the associated acupoints and reflexes of Ki 27, Con 22 and hand reflexes 28 and 18. They should be finger pad massaged for about 1 minute each. It is these four points that are very good to use on a regular basis by the patient. They should be instructed in their use.
5. The lung meridian great point of Lu 7 is now massaged for 2–3 minutes. The patient should be feeling a good deal better by now.
6. Balance the general energy across the Sheng cycle of the five elements.

Acute bronchitis

Acute bronchitis may be accompanied by pain and discomfort, dyspnoea, wheezing and chest tightness. The treatment is as follows (see Figure 4.3):

1. The associated meridian is the *lung* meridian, to be stroked against the flow of energy two or three times.
2. Hold the local point Lu 1 and distal point Lu 9 until an energy balance is reached. This can take up to 3 minutes if the symptoms are more sub-acute.
3. Massage point Bl 13 for at least 2 minutes. This point is found on the 'inner bladder line' over the transverse process of T3. It is best performed whilst the patient is comfortably sitting. Other very useful special points are hand reflex points 28 and 29 plus the lung areas on the soles of the feet. The latter need to be massaged very gently, almost caressed. Please remember that the lungs are composed of very delicate membranous tissue, and the massage of the associated reflex should be equally as delicate – it will pay dividends in the long run if this simple message is adhered to.
4. The great point of the Lung meridian, Lu 7 should now be gently stimulated for up to 3 minutes.
5. Finally balance the body's general energy around the Sheng cycle.

The common cold

It is a well-known saying that 'a cold gets better in one week with treatment or in seven days without treatment'. It is true that the symptoms of a cold will probably run their course whatever is done to try and change them. Millions of pounds are spent on medicines to attempt to ease the situation. Some of them work; some of them do not. It seems to me that the best possible way of attempting to rid the body of the pathogens that cause the common cold are to strengthen the immune system. This can be achieved by improving the energy system by means of acupressure. Treatment on the immune system is discussed in the next chapter, but here is discussed the treatment of the acute symptoms of rhinitis and coryza. It is essential, though, that other treatment is also tried. This includes taking vitamin C in high doses (about 3 g per day), zinc, selenium and increasing the intake of water three-fold. Also, cut out sugar, caffeine, fats and all synthetic foods – the body is attempting to cleanse itself of impurities and

Figure 4.3 Points used in acute bronchitis.

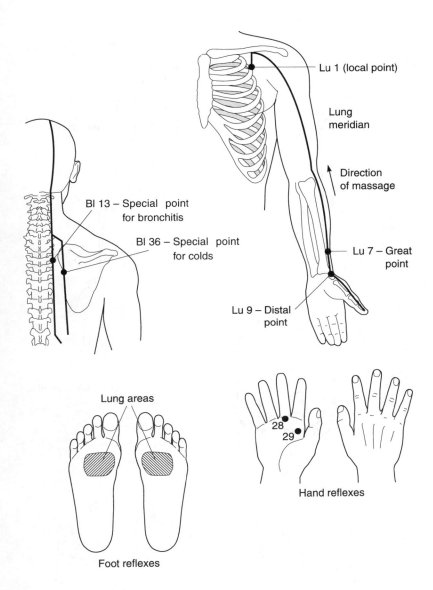

Lu 1 (local point)

Lung meridian

Direction of massage

Bl 13 – Special point for bronchitis

Bl 36 – Special point for colds

Lu 7 – Great point

Lu 9 – Distal point

Lung areas

28
29

Hand reflexes

Foot reflexes

it will not be helped if rubbish food is eaten. The following acupressure treatments should be followed (see Figure 4.4):

1. Stroke the large intestine meridian against the flow of energy, from head to hand, three times, followed by the lung meridian from hand to chest three times. This can be done over clothes if necessary.
2. There is no clear local point, but Ki 27 makes an excellent all-round point. Stimulate this point for a couple of minutes. This brings energy to the area and starts to energize the thyroid as well. Also stimulate LI 4 for a minute and finally balance the energy between the two. This may take up to 3 minutes. If the symptoms are purely localized to the nose, the local point can be LI 20.
3. The patient can then be instructed to self-treat using the hand reflexes 17, 33 and 34. These tend to boost the immune system. The face

Figure 4.4 Points used for common cold.

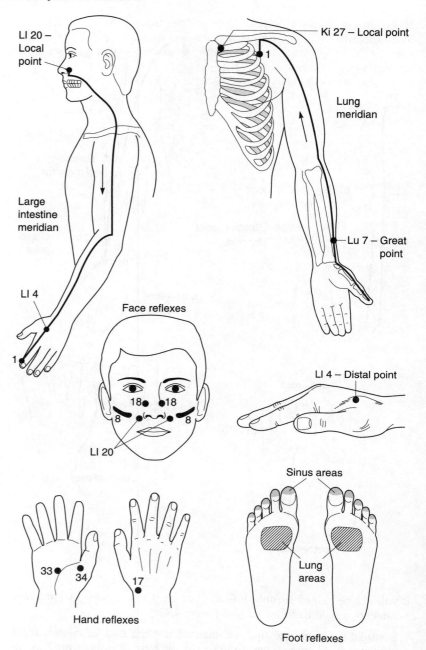

reflexes 8 and the area along the inferior border of the zygoma should now be massaged, gently at first and becoming deeper as discomfort allows. These facial reflex points are especially useful in blocked sinuses and nasal cavities. The lung and sinus reflex areas on the feet can also be massaged.

4.   Stimulate the great point of the lung meridian Lu 7 for anything up to 3 minutes.

5.   Finally, balance the general body energy around the Sheng cycle.

Procedures 1–4 may be repeated up to three times a day. It really does make the difference of being able to resume normal activities by easing some of the nasty symptoms that a common cold can give. The foregoing treatment may also be carried out on influenza symptoms, although more of the immune system boosting procedures needs to be done.

Acute skin conditions

What does one do to treat an acute flare up of eczema, pruritus or dermatitis? These acute conditions can be very unpleasant and can prove to be very difficult to treat. There are often some side effects if topical cortisone creams are applied. Some non-acupressure methods that I have found work very well in easing the burning and excoriating symptoms are as follows:

(a) Cut an apple in half and rub the cut bit on the locally affected area for up to 2 minutes. Alternatively, eat the apple and rub the apple core on the affected skin.
(b) Gently massage some Milk of Magnesia (or Cream of Magnesia) onto the skin. Do not do this if the skin is cut. The magnesia is very cooling but soon turns powdery, so needs to washed off with cold water afterwards.
(c) Tincture of marigold, or better still some proprietary branded calendula lotion or ointment. There is also some excellent herbal and low potency homoeopathic skin ointments that can be easily obtained from the pharmacy.

It must be understood that on no account will the various lotions and acupressure described below treat the cause of the skin eruption. Aetiology of skin conditions are numerous and outside the scope of this book. The following acupressure techniques may be employed (see Figure 4.5):

1. The associated meridians are the stomach, lung and large intestine. This is because skin conditions are often attributed to eating faulty food (stomach), the skin is often called the third lung (lung), and a meridian of excretion is needed (large intestine). These meridians need to be stroked against the flow of energy three times each.
2. It is obviously impossible to have a local point if one is talking holistically. Never, ever use a local point that is over the area of skin eruption. Remember that eczema is a symptom of expression of the whole body, and where it is on the body is often immaterial. The 'local' point that has been carefully chosen is Con 14, which is found distal to the xiphoid process. This point is said to be the physical counterpart of the solar plexus chakra and as such has influence on some skin conditions. This point needs to be stimulated (not harshly) for 2 minutes. LI 4 then needs to be stimulated for a minute before the two points are balanced with each other until a change of influence is felt. Please note that LI 4 is not to be stimulated in pregnancy or in the first 2 days of menstruation. If this is the case, LI 11 may be used as an alternative.

Figure 4.5 Points used for skin conditions.

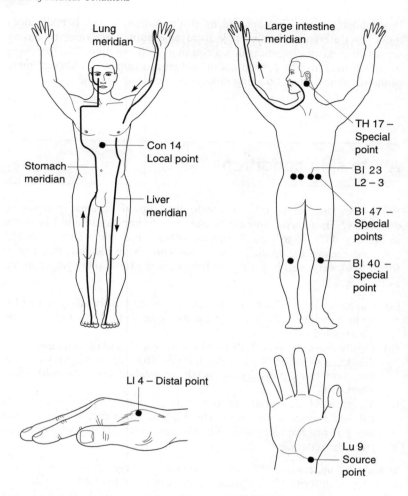

3. There are three special points and each has a different influence. TH 17, situated behind the lobe of the ear, is an excellent point to be used when there is much redness and heat. Bl 40 is a traditional point in treating skin conditions with acupuncture, and it seems to be one of those occasions where it is just as effective with pressure. It dispels damp and removes heat from blood. Stimulate the two Bl 40 points for at least 3 minutes. The combination points of Bl 23 and Bl 47 are to be found at the level of L2–L3. These points are usually used in improving the general energy of the body and also in the liberation of adrenaline. They seem to work very well, however, in treating skin conditions.

4. The source point of the lung meridian, Lu 9, is the best point to use to improve the general energy quality of the skin.

5. Finally, balance the body energy using the Sheng cycle.

Please do not expect miracles to occur with this method, but you should be pleasantly surprised at how useful acupressure can be in treating skin conditions.

Ear, nose and throat conditions

Earache

There is nothing more miserable than earache, especially in children. Below is an acupressure routine that takes less than 5 minutes that should ease most earache pain. The obvious exception to this is when accident or injury affects the internal ear, or when there is much bacterial or viral infection. This procedure should ease the pain whilst other treatment will tackle the infection (see Figure 4.6).

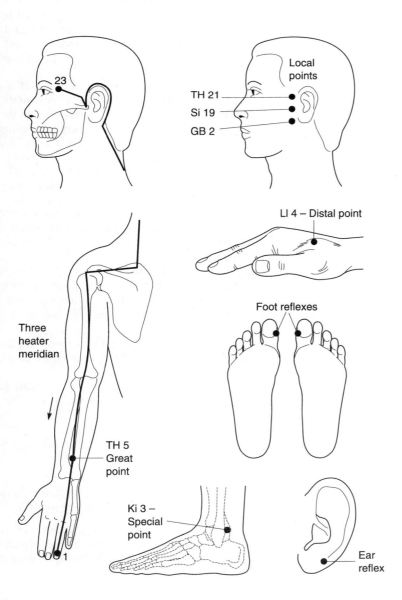

Figure 4.6 Points used in earche.

1. The associated meridian is the three heater. This is partly because the meridian passes around the ear and partly because it has been found to be the most effective. The meridian should be stroked three times against the flow of energy from ear to hand. Be careful when stroking around the ear that it does not cause too much discomfort.

2. There are three local points – TH 21, Si 19 and GB 2. The location and numbering of these 'three little maids' have been learnt by innumerable acupuncture students. When using acupressure, they can all be used together. It is usually possible to place the ring, middle and index fingers on these points with the patient lying down and the arm supported. If, in the case of a child it is too painful to keep the finger pads *in situ*, place them on exactly the same points on the good ear! This sounds a little far-fetched, but it works – it is parallel acupressure in action! If both ears are painful, the local points will have to be dispensed with. In this case just stimulate LI 4. If the fingers can be placed by the ear, balance energy between the local points and LI 4. You will have to hold for about 2 minutes until the pain starts to ease. Do not stimulate LI 4 in pregnancy or in the first 2 days of menstruation.

3. There are three useful special points, two reflex points and an acupoint. Ki 3 is situated posterior to the medial malleolus next to the Achilles tendon. Traditional Chinese medicine philosophy couples the kidney with the ear, so it is no surprise that one of the very best points for earache should be on the kidney meridian. Stimulating massage for about 2 minutes is needed on this point. Do not stimulate in pregnancy. There is a very good reflex point, would you believe, in the ear. The ear reflexes are sometimes forgotten at the expense of using body points but where they are valuable, they have been included. The ear point is one such point. It needs to be pressed with the thumb and forefinger opposing each other either side of the pinna for about 2 minutes. I have seen painful earaches clear by just using this point. The final special point is the ear reflex on the foot, which is situated on the medial aspect of the great toe. Experience has shown that there is a much better success rate in using this particular point than the classical ear reflex areas underneath the toes. These points need to be gently stimulated for a few seconds and then just held for up to 3 minutes.

4. The discomfort should be gone by now, but to prevent its return, the great point in earache, TH 5, should be stimulated, on both forearms, for 2 minutes.

5. It is not always applicable to balance the general energy, especially in children who may have just returned to sleep, but where possible, please do it.

Conjunctivitis

The treatment of conjunctivitis and other localized inflammatory conditions of the eye answer very well to acupressure (see Figure 4.7).

1. Stroke the bladder meridian against the flow of energy from the outer border of the little toe, up the back of the leg and back, around the head and to the forehead. It goes without saying that the therapist cannot stroke as far as the inner canthus of the eye.

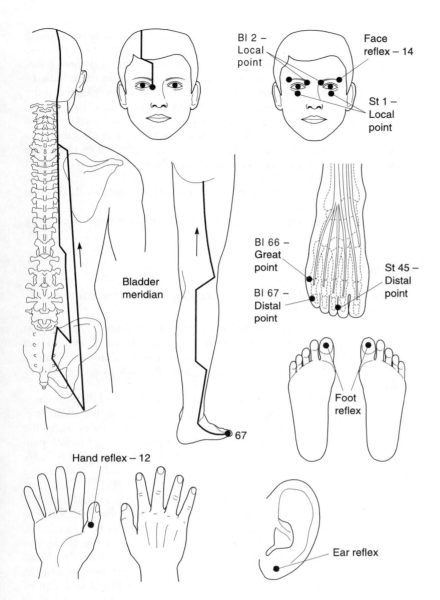

Figure 4.7 Points used in conjunctivitis.

2. There are two possible local points – Bl 2 and St 1. Because of the inflammatory nature of this condition, it is not always possible to use local points. The alternative is to use the local points of the other eye or to just use the distal points. Where it is possible to use both sets of points, please do so. The distal points are Bl 67 and St 45. This is a classic example of using energy along a meridian from the end point to the Tsing point as a way of drawing excess energy, heat and inflammation away from one end of the meridian. When balancing the two points, the patient should be in the sitting position with the knees bent up, otherwise the therapist will have to have extended arms in order to perform this technique. When using just the distal points, have the patient comfortably long sitting or lying down. Both distal points

can be treated at the same time and they need to be held for about 5 minutes.

3. Special reflex points are situated on the ear, face, foot and hand. Possibly the most effective is the ear point, situated in the middle of the pinna of the ear, closely followed by the foot reflex, situated at the 'pituitary' point in the middle of the great toe. Since attending a course in Reflexology and Language of the Feet with Chris Stormer I have found that this 'alternative' eye point seems to be more effective than the more popular area under the great toe. The other reflex points are hand reflex 12 on the side of the thumb and face reflex 14 on the upper outer border of the eyebrow.

4. Next massage the great point for this condition, which is Bl 66 – do this for up to 3 minutes.

5. Balance the general energy by balancing points around the Sheng cycle.

Toothache

The treatment of toothache with acupressure can be very effective (see Figure 4.8).

1. There are two associated meridians depending on whether there is pain in the upper or lower mouth. Use the large intestine meridian for upper mouth pain and the stomach meridian in lower mouth discomfort. These meridians should be stroked against the flow of energy two or three times.

2. In upper mouth discomfort, the local point is LI 20 and distal point is LI 1. When self-treating, point LI 1 may be used in isolation. It is especially effective when waiting to see the dentist (plus using the appropriate points for anticipation!). When treating lower mouth pain there is a choice of local points – St 4 or St 6. The distal point is St 36. Be careful not to massage this point too enthusiastically: it can cause nausea and vomiting.

3. There are three very useful reflex areas – on the ear, hand and foot. The ear reflex is positioned on the anterior aspect of the pinna. It should be squeezed quite hard between thumb and forefinger for up to a minute. Students of mine have often observed that squeezing the ear in this manner works because it produces a counter-irritant effect. The Hand reflex point 30 seems to work very well in self-treatment whilst the foot reflexes on the pads of the toes are very effective if time can be spent on them. It is often the case, though, in toothache that an instant miracle needs to occur.

4. The great point to use is LI 4. As the reader is now aware, it is the most effective distal point in acupressure for the relief of pain in the face, head, shoulders and chest. It should though, on no account be used in pregnancy and during menstruation. The point should be gently massaged for up to 3 minutes or until the last trace of pain has gone.

5. There is usually no need to balance the general energy in this very localized condition.

Nosebleeds (epistaxis)

Nosebleeds can be both frustrating and embarrassing. They may be caused by stress, high blood pressure or as a result of an old mechanical irritation

Figure 4.8 Points used in toothache.

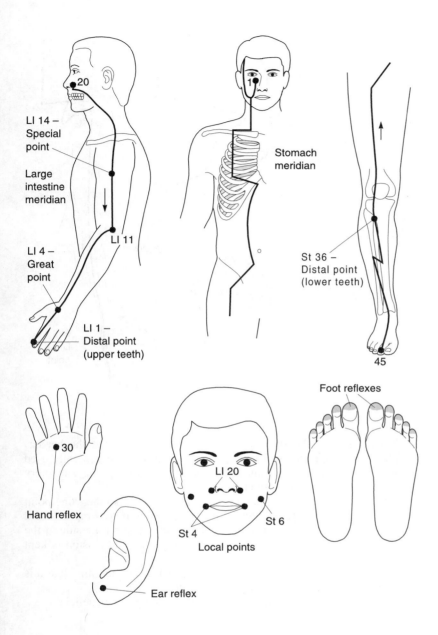

to the inner septum that has caused some scabbing. The treatment of stress and high blood pressure will be discussed later in the book, so the following procedure is effective in treating nosebleeds as a first aid measure (see Figure 4.9):

1. The associated meridian is the small intestine. This should be stroked against the flow of energy, from ear to little finger, three or four times.
2. There are two local points – Gov 26 and St 3. Gov 26 is situated just below the nose on the upper lip in the midline. It is best used as just a local point without needing to do any energy balancing work. It is a very useful first aid point in that it can also be used in revival from fainting. Stimulate this point for up to 5 minutes or until the bleeding

Figure 4.9 Points used in nosebleeds.

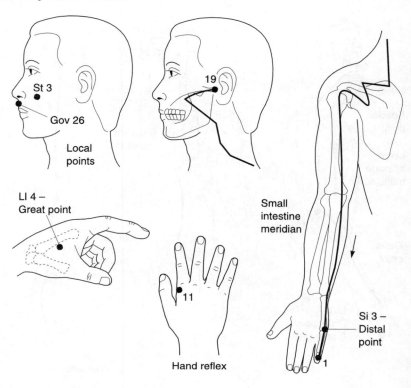

has stopped. Make sure the person is relaxed and that the head is placed in extension. St 3 and the distal point Si 3 are generally used when someone else is administering the treatment. They are very effective but can take some time.

3. The best special point is hand reflex 11, which is also the same point as LI 3. A good tip in order to stop nosebleeds is to wrap a folded handkerchief tightly over the knuckles of the hand on the side of the nosebleed, so that it affects both Si 3 and LI 3. The tension is kept going by clenching the fist.

4. The great point is once again, our friend LI 4. Do not stimulate this point in pregnancy or in early menstruation.

5. General energy balancing via the Sheng cycle will be beneficial.

Sinusitis and hay fever symptoms

The pain of sinusitis can be one of the most acutely traumatic experiences. It is caused by inflammation of the mucous membrane linings of one or more of the three sinus cavities in the skull. There is then a swelling of the membranes and mucous cannot escape. (See Figure 4.10.)

1. The associated meridian is the Lung channel. Traditional Chinese medicine dictates that the nasal passages are governed by energy that serves the lungs and skin. It needs to be stroked against the flow of energy two or three times.

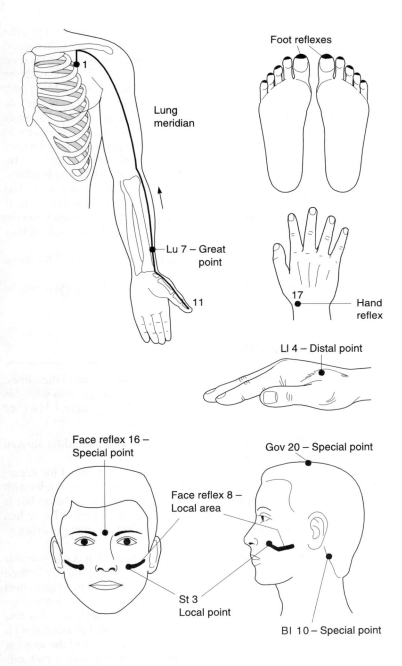

Figure 4.10 Points used in sinusitis and hayfever.

Foot reflexes

Lung meridian

Lu 7 – Great point

11

17

Hand reflex

LI 4 – Distal point

Face reflex 16 – Special point

Gov 20 – Special point

Face reflex 8 – Local area

St 3 Local point

BI 10 – Special point

2. There are two local points, St 3 and face reflex area 8. These two can obviously be used together as they are adjacent to each other. They should be firmly massaged with finger or thumb pad kneading for about 2 minutes. The pressure of the massage should be guided by the amount of discomfort. The distal point is LI 4. The energy balance between these two points is extremely effective in initially easing the discomfort and allowing relaxation of the membranes to take place. The energy balance should be held for anything up to 6 minutes.

3. There are five special points for sinusitis to be used as a back up to the previous procedure. They are Gov 20, Extra 1, Bl 10, foot reflexes and hand reflex 17. They are each used for different effects. Gov 20 is used to ease the sensation of 'fullness' and heaviness in the head. With the patient lying supine the therapist is positioned at their head. Place both hands gently on the top of the head with both middle fingers either side of Gov 20. Gently press down into the skull and part the hands away from each other at the same time. This may take up to 10 minutes to have the desired effect. Extra 1 (or facial reflex point 16) may be used for its calming effect either by itself or in combination with Gov 16. Bl 10 is used to ease the tension at the back of the neck and head that so often accompanies acute sinusitis. Hand reflex 17 is a first class reflex point that can be used in self-treatment. If the reflex point is tender, it should be used. The foot reflexes on the tips of each toe are useful when treated in conjunction with a full foot reflexology treatment.
4. Finally, stimulate the great point of the lung meridian, Lu 7 for about 3 minutes.
5. The balancing of the body's general energy via the Sheng cycle will be most beneficial.

Sore throat and tonsillitis

Nearly everyone gets a sore throat and tonsillitis at some time in their lives. Although acupressure cannot deal with the infection that persists with this condition, it can be beneficial in helping the discomfort (Figure 4.11). (See the next chapter for the treatment of immune system deficiencies.)

1. The associated meridian is the lung channel. This should be stroked against the flow of energy two or three times.
2. The local point is Con 22, which is situated in the centre of the supra-sternal fossa just above the sternal notch. This point is very tender with sore throats, so care must be taken. It can be used in isolation but is best used in the balancing of energy with the distal point LI 4. When using this combination of points, the patient must be sitting or lying as it could make them feel light-headed.
3. There are a number of special points that can be used. It is not essential to use all of them – they each have a different action. Ki 27, located under the medial end of the clavicle, may be stimulated to relieve chest congestion, tightness of the chest and coughing. Gov 14, located on the spine between C7 and T1 is used to relax the neck muscles that become so tight in the person trying to protect the pain associated with tonsillitis. Bl 38, located between the shoulder blades and the spine at the level of T4–T5, is used to clear the bronchial passages and aids breathing. There are two hand reflexes – points 29 and 6. Point 29 is used when symptoms are more severe, point 6 is used in mild sore throats. The foot reflexes may be used to great effect either in isolation or in combination with the lung reflected area. The best special point is Ki 3. This point is located between the medial malleolus and the Achilles tendon. It is particularly effective when treating a raging sore throat. The ear reflex may be squeezed as part of a self-help procedure.
4. Finally, the great point of the Lung meridian, Lu 7 should be stimulated for at least 3 minutes.

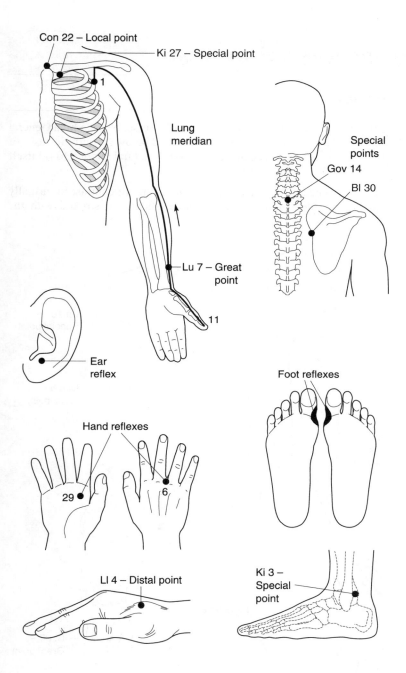

Figure 4.11 Points used in sore throats.

5.   It is very beneficial to balance the general energy via the Sheng cycle.

The non-acupressure advice in the treatment of sore throats is as follows:

(a) Drink plenty of bland fluids.
(b) Drink hot honey and lemon drink.
(c) Chew a piece of ginger and let it dissolve at the back of the throat.
(d) Aspirin gargles are very beneficial.
(e) Cut out sugar and dairy produce in the diet.

Gastro-intestinal conditions

Diarrhoea

Severe diarrhoea of unknown origin must, of course, be seen by a General Practitioner. The treatment procedure described below is useful in cases of food poisoning. Diarrhoea occurs as the body's natural attempt to rid itself of the toxins. (See Figure 4.12.)

1. The associated meridian is the large intestine. In contrast to virtually all other acute conditions, the channel should be stroked with the

Figure 4.12 Points used in diarrhoea.

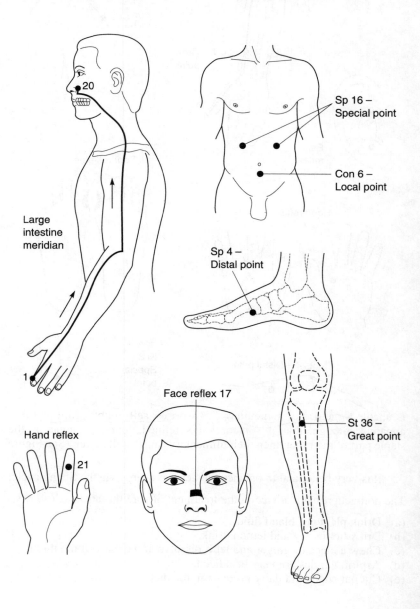

energy flow, i.e. from forefinger to nose. This should be performed at least six times at each session of treatment and treatment should be done at least once an hour or until the symptoms subside. Although diarrhoea is acute, painful and a very 'here and now' situation, it is essentially a question of balancing the body's fluids. In all cases of fluid imbalance, the condition can be regarded as being Yin, therefore needs to be stimulated.

2. The local point used is Con 6, which is situated in the midline 1.5 cun inferior to the umbilicus. In esoteric philosophy, this point is said to be the physical counterpart of the sacral chakra, which is the chakra associated with fluid retention. This point should be stimulated for about 2 minutes. The distal point is Sp 4, situated just distal to the first metatarsal. This point is used in most cases of discomfort with the abdominal region and seems to the perfect choice as a distal point. It should be stimulated for 2 minutes before an energy balance is attempted with Con 6. This part of the treatment will best deal with the water imbalance.

3. There are three special points – Sp 16, face reflex 17 and hand reflex 21. Sp 16 is located below the edge of the rib cage 0.5 cun from the vertical nipple line. It seems to be a good point in relieving the many symptoms of diarrhoea, including cramping and bloating. It is also a good point in the treatment of stomach ulcers. Face reflex no. 17 is a broad band area situated on the bridge of the nose. It may be used in self-help and is particularly useful in the pain of diarrhoea. Hand reflex 21 is located in the middle of the palmar aspect of the forefinger. It is another point that is useful in the pain associated with diarrhoea.

4. The great point used at the end of the treatment is St 36. This point will probably be quite tender to the touch. It should be stimulated for anything up to 3 minutes. Do not over-stimulate this point, however, as it can cause nausea and sometimes vomiting.

5. Finally, balance the general energy via the Sheng cycle.

Constipation

Although not strictly an acute condition, it is placed in this section because it is generally treated on an acute level and not, as it should be, as a chronic energy imbalance. Although it may be considered that constipation occurs as a result of faulty eating or the side effects of some drug medication, it mostly happens as a result of a psychosomatic imbalance where the person is unable to get rid of something, e.g. worries, self-doubts, guilt etc. It is apparent, though, that if someone eats refined flour and sugar as the staple part of their diet, then their alimentary canals will suffer. (See Figure 4.13.)

1. The associated meridian is the large intestine channel. The meridian needs to be stroked against the flow of energy several times (up to a dozen) before proceeding to the next part of the treatment.

2. The local point used is Con 6 (as in diarrhoea) and the distal point is St 36. These two points need to be stimulated for about a minute before an energy balance is attempted between the two.

3. There are three useful reflexes that can be used in constipation – on the hand, foot and face. The face reflex no. 21 is situated in the midline on

Figure 4.13 Points used in constipation.

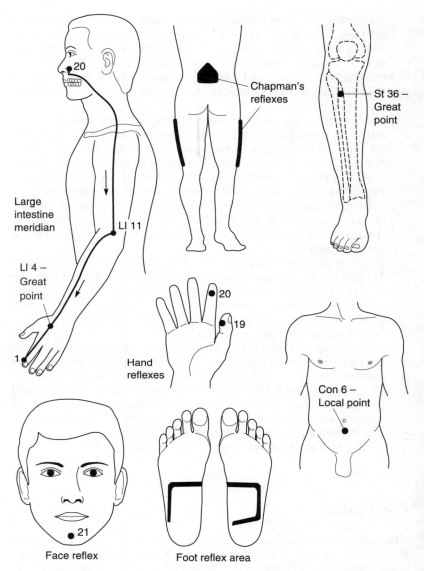

the chin and is generally used for the pain associated with this condition. Hand reflexes nos 19 and 20 may be used in self-treatment on a regular basis to help with peristaltic movement. The foot reflexes are most useful. They should be massaged with some degree of gusto and enthusiasm, with the exception of when the practitioner knows that there is also some other associated large bowel disease such as Crohn's disease or chronic irritable bowel syndrome. In these cases, the reflex should be treated gently. In this section of the treatment, there is a variation to all the other acute conditions. Because, as has been stated previously, constipation is really a chronic condition, Chapman's reflex massage is introduced here. Chapman's reflexes are useful in all conditions where there is sluggishness, induration and stiffness. The associated areas of the large intestine lie along the course of the ilio-tibial tract on the outer aspect of the thighs and a large area around the lower lumbar spine. Warn the patient that these areas can be very painful. Added to this is the fact that one of the best ways to treat these areas is with connective tissue massage. This is, by far, the most stimulating massage that one can do. It is generally worth it, though, as it is a very effective treatment.

4. The great point used is LI 4. This should be stimulated for up to 5 minutes. Please do not use this point in pregnancy or in the initial stages of menstruation. Use LI 11 as an alternate.
5. Finally, balance the body's energies via the Sheng cycle.

Gastritis, indigestion and nausea

It is possible to clump these three conditions together as the points used in acupressure are the same (see Figure 4.14).

1. The associated meridian is the stomach channel. This needs to be stroked against the flow of energy, from fourth toe to eye three or four times.
2. The local point in gastritis and indigestion is Con 12. This point is located just below the xiphoid process in the midline. An alternative local point in gastritis is St 21, which is located 2 cun lateral to the midline, 4 cun above the umbilicus. On no account should these points be stimulated in acute gastritis – the pain will be made worse. The points should be sedated for anything up to 5 minutes. When the therapist is sure that the heat has been dispelled from the area, the distal point of Sp 4 may be introduced. Energy balancing between these two points may take up to 3 or 4 minutes.
3. There are seven special points that may be considered in these conditions. Bl 23 is located by the transverse processes between L2 and L3. Stimulation on this point will help with indigestion and abdominal pain. It is a very versatile point in that it helps with improvement of general energy and with anxiety in that it helps to improve the function of the adrenal glands in the production of adrenaline. GB 24 is located on the vertical nipple line in the seventh intercostal space. It is often a very tender point. It is used mostly in acute indigestion due to eating too much or eating too much fatty food, hence its use in gall bladder colic and hepatitis. The hand reflexes 19 and 35 are useful in self-treatment and the stomach area reflex of the feet is also very useful. When using the foot reflexes at this level, the diaphragm points may also be treated so as to cause relaxation in the abdomen in general, thus aiding the healing process. Face reflex 15 is used in acute gastritis and nausea. The best point to use in nausea, though, is P 6. This point is located 2 cun proximal to the anterior wrist crease. It has wide ranging uses in many types of nausea that are caused by motion sickness, gastritis, drug intolerance or in pregnancy. The point should be pressed quite hard and stimulated at a slow rhythm for up to 3 or 4 minutes. There has been much discussion about the use of the so-called 'sea bands'. These are elastic bands containing a small magnet that is strategically placed just above the wrist and supposed to cure sea-sickness. I have always been of the opinion that

Figure 4.14 Points used in gastritis.

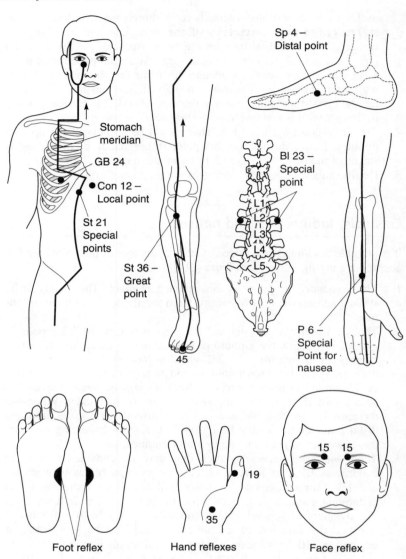

massaging P6 could save a great deal of money.

4.   The great point in all symptoms associated with the stomach, indigestion and nausea is St 36. This is probably the second most important point in acupressure, next to LI 4. It is so useful in very many conditions. Be careful not to massage it with too much enthusiasm – it could make the nausea worse. If this occurs, just touch the point with light pressure for about 5 minutes – it works wonders!

5.   Finally, balance the general body's energy by balancing around the Sheng cycle.

Genito-urinary conditions

Cystitis

There is just one condition to consider in the section of genito-urinary conditions, but one that causes absolute misery to its unfortunate sufferers. (See Figure 4.15.)

1. The associated meridian, as one would expect, is the bladder channel. This should be stroked against the flow of energy four or five times.

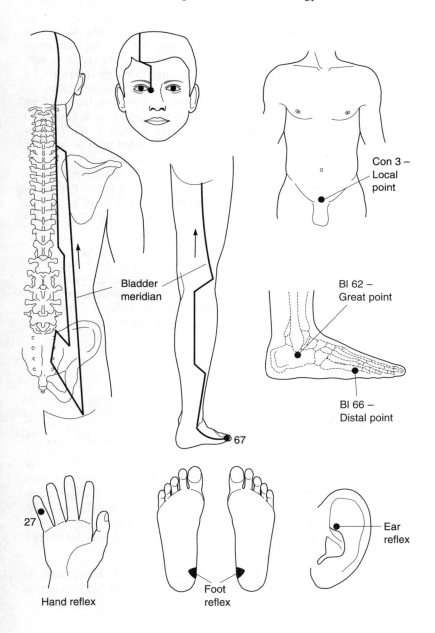

Figure 4.15 Points used in cystitis.

Try a deeper pressure around the outside of the foot and the small of the back.

2. The local point in cystitis is Con 3. This point is situated 4 cun below the umbilicus. Be careful not to press too hard on this point in cases of very acute pain – your patient will not appreciate it. The best approach is to gently increase the amount of pressure on this point over a period of a few minutes. Whilst holding this point, the other hand could be locating and treating Bl 66. This is probably the best distal point in the treatment of cystitis, although Bl 64 runs it close. Following this balance, the patient should have much less pain, but using the special points will enhance the treatment and create a significant improvement.

3. The special points in cystitis are located in the hand, foot and ear. Hand reflex 27 is a truly wonderful reflected point that may be used in self-treatment. The patient should be encouraged to massage this point for a couple of minutes at least every half hour. The foot reflexes may also be of great benefit either in self-treatment or with the help of a therapist. When using these reflexes, try not to be in a hurry about it. The best way is to just touch the bilateral points with the forearms supported on the couch for anything up to 10 minutes. Your client will love you forever. The other reflex point is located in the anterior section of the antihelix part of the ear. It is a useful point in analysis and treatment of the more acute episodes of cystitis.

4. To finish this part of the treatment, massage the great point of the bladder meridian, Bl 62. It is located just distal to the lateral malleolus. It needs to be gently massaged for about 2 minutes. If, in massaging Bl 62, the discomfort returns, try just holding the point gently. This usually does the trick.

5. Now balance around the Sheng cycle.

It is essential, in cystitis, that the patient drinks about three times their normal intake of water or bland fluid. Do not have sugar, red meats, dairy produce or citrus fruits. There are many herbal and homoeopathic remedies that can be tried. Possibly the best is homoeopathic cantharis. Take this in a 6 or 30 potency every 10 minutes for up to six doses, then hourly until the symptoms subside.

Gynaecological conditions

Hot flushes

Hot flushes represent one of the more unpleasant side effects of the menopause. They occur when oestrogen levels suddenly decrease with age. The production of oestrogen is regulated by the pituitary gland, which is situated adjacent to the hypothalamus which regulates the body's temperature control. (See Figure 4.16.)

1. The associated meridian is the three heater channel. This should be stroked against the flow of energy three or four times. Make sure that the area of the channel around the ear is given special attention.

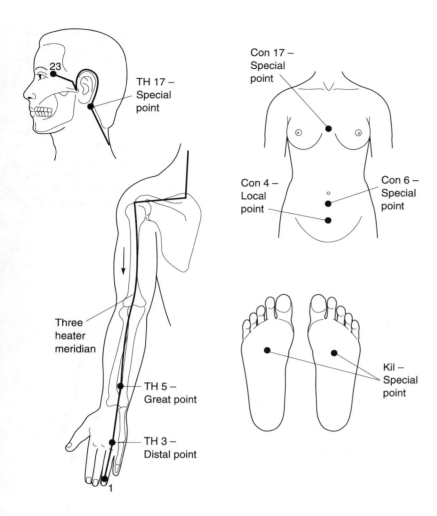

Figure 4.16 Points used in hot flushes.

2. The local point in this and many other gynaecological conditions is Con 4. This point is located 3 cun inferior to the umbilicus in the midline. The point should be mildly stimulated for about 1 minute before the other hand locates the Distal point TH 3. This point is located on the posterior aspect of the hand, between the fourth and fifth metacarpals and proximal to the metacarpo-phalangeal joint. These two points should be energy balanced until a change of emphasis occurs.

3. The special points used in this condition are Con 6, Con 17 and Ki 1. Con 6 can be treated when there are other symptoms of the menopause, i.e. swollen ankles, headaches, clumsiness, forgetfulness etc. Con 17 may be used when anxiety or nervousness is present. Regular hot flushes can prove to be very disruptive. This can often bring about anxious and nervous sensations, especially if they are severe. Con 17 should be used if these symptoms are present (see Chapter 6 for the treatment of other psychosomatic disorders). When there is anxiety, but also light-headedness and fainting sensations, the point of choice is Ki 1, on the soles of the feet. This is a useful first aid point that can be used in many similar circumstances.

4. The great point in this condition is TH 5. This point is located 2 cun proximal to the posterior wrist crease. It should be given mild stimulation for about 3 or 4 minutes, or until the heat subsides. Patients should be encouraged to use this point freely in self-help.
5. Balancing energy around the Sheng cycle will help.

Period pain and morning sickness

Period pain or 'cramps' can prove to be more than just a regular inconvenience. Some women suffer a great deal of pain. Full details of how to treat this will be given in the next chapter but below are details of how to deal with acute discomfort at that 'time of the month'. (See Figure 4.17.)

Figure 4.17 Points used in period pain.

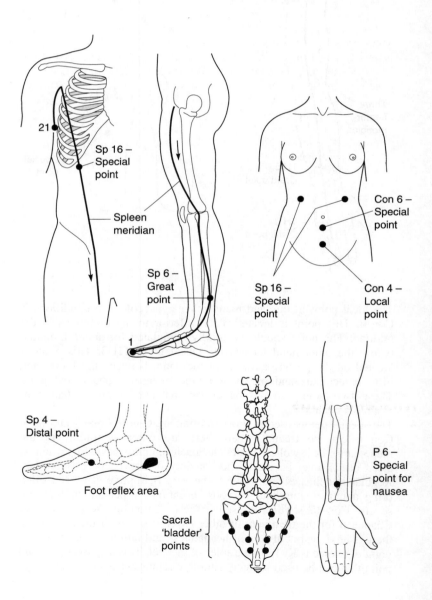

1. The associated meridian is the spleen channel. It should be stroked against the flow of energy three or four times prior to the main part of the treatment. Emphasis should be placed on the area of the spleen meridian from the great toe to the knee.
2. The local point that was discussed in the section on hot flushes is Con 4. This point should be gently massaged for 2 or 3 minutes. This should take the 'edge' off the pain. Then make contact with Sp 4, on the instep of the foot, and gently massage both points in unison, until a warm glow is felt under the fingers. This may take up to 4 minutes.
3. There are five special points available to help in the treatment of this condition. Con 6 has been mentioned before – this is especially useful in more chronic cases and where there is some ankle or abdominal swelling. Sp 16 is located on the inferior aspect of the rib cage between the eighth and ninth rib cartilage, half a cun from the vertical nipple line. It is very useful in generalized abdominal cramps (including hiccups) so tends to relax the whole of the abdominal area. There are several bladder meridian points situated in the sacrum. They generally lie in the various sacral fossae and in the sacro-iliac joint. These should be massaged (with oil) with heavy stimulation for a couple of minutes. They tend to release the tension around the area which all helps in the healing process. The best reflex point to use in this condition is the foot reflex. It is situated on the medial aspect of the heels. These two points should be held until the pain eases, which after doing the previous work should not take too long. The specific point to use in the treatment of morning sickness is P6. This point was described in the previous section on nausea.
4. The great point in this and other gynaecological conditions is Sp 6. This point is located 3 cun superior to the medial malleolus and just behind the tibial border. It is one of the most used points in the whole of acupressure. It should be massaged for three minutes or so, or until the pain subsides.
5. Finally, balance the body's energy via the Sheng cycle.

A non-acupressure treatment of period pain is to take homoeopathic Mag Phos 6. This is easily obtained from a chemist or health store. It should be taken every 10 minutes for an hour, or until the discomfort eases, then once every two hours during the day. Keep the lower abdomen warm and drink lots of hot chamomile tea.

Miscellaneous

Fainting

This can occur at any time and for a variety of reasons, and it is best to know how to handle the situation. It probably occurs less within the rooms of an acupressure and reflextherapy practitioner than with an acupuncturist, for obvious reasons. (See Figure 4.18.)

1. There is no specific associated meridian.
2. As fainting constitutes a first aid situation, it is essential that the most effective point be tried first, once this has worked, the other points may

Figure 4.18 Points used in fainting.

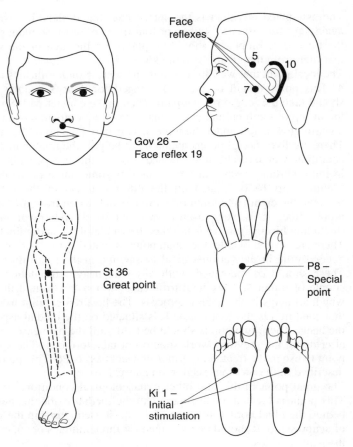

be used to supplement the treatment. Ki 1 is the treatment of choice. The two points should be gently stimulated until there are signs of recovery. The treatment can be done through socks and tights (but not shoes). Ki 1 is one of the best first aid points in shock and convulsions; in fainting it must be stimulated, not just held.

3.   There are five other special points that can be tried. P8 is located in the centre of the hand and is a good substitute for Ki 1. In subtle anatomy terms, P8 is the hand chakra and Ki 1 represents the foot chakra. These are also associated with the crown chakra – so there is an energy link. It may be much easier to access this point than by grovelling on the floor taking shoes off. The face has three reflected areas that can be useful – points 5, 7 and area 10. Point 5 should be stimulated after an obvious shock to the patient. This point is efficient in improving the blood flow to the brain. Point 7 is used when the cause of the fainting is low blood pressure, and the area around the ear, point 10, should be used when there is high blood pressure. Massage should be very gentle, as this is a very sensitive area of the head. By far the best special point is Gov 26. This point is situated on the top lip, just underneath the nose. It should be massaged on a regular basis if the patient is prone to having 'light' heads. If in doubt, always consult the General Practitioner, as there could be a more sinister underlying cause that would need to be investigated.

4. The great point to use after the patient has recovered is St 36. This is one of the main 'energy' points on the body and can help accelerate the recovery process.
5. It will be advantageous to balance the energy via the Sheng cycle once the patient has recovered sufficiently.

Pain

This chapter concludes by discussing how to treat pain. For many practitioners and therapists, treating pain is the 'be all and end all' of successful therapy. It is true, of course, that the majority of patients who seek treatment are suffering from some kind of pain, and their reason for attending is for someone else to ease their discomfort. The therapist has to walk a tightrope, on one hand the pain has to be eased; on the other hand, the cause of the condition should be addressed. As has been stated before, if the cause is not treated, the symptoms, which include pain, will reoccur at a later date. There is no easy answer to this dilemma. The solution is often to be found in the conscience of the practitioner. Bad practitioners merely placate and suppress, whereas good practitioners treat the whole person. The latter is what should be occurring in the whole of medicine, but sadly it is not. There are bad practitioners in therapy, just as there are bad builders and electricians.

This section deals with acute pain, but the points described will also be of great use in treating chronic pain. The golden rule in treating acute and sensitive pain is to initially *sedate*. In other words, the acupoints and reflexes are gently pressed, massaged and held – they are not stimulated to any degree as this could make the pain worse. When the pain is either sub-acute or chronic, the initial emphasis is on *stimulation* of the points. This can either be performed with deep pressure circling of the points, as in shiatsu, or by quick rotational movements, as in Tuina. After the initial sedation or stimulation of the relevant points, the treatment of the condition should proceed with *energy balancing*. This procedure has been adequately described in a previous chapter. It seems to me that with this all-round approach to acupressure and reflextherapy, the philosophy of how pain relief is achieved by touch can be explained. Pain relief of acute conditions with sedation may be explained by balancing superficial and aura body energies, and pain relief of chronic conditions with stimulation is explained by the endorphin release theory. This and the other theories of pain relief will be discussed in Chapter 5.

Figure 4.19 shows the various pain-relieving points. There are, of course, several more points that are used in pain relief, but those mentioned below seem to be the most effective.

LI 4

As has been mentioned before, LI 4 is probably the most used point in acupressure. It is such a versatile point. It is situated between the first and second metacarpals when the thumb is fully extended. The Chinese for LI 4 is 'Hegu' or 'Hoku'. These words are translated as 'the great eliminator'.

Figure 4.19 Points used in pain relief.

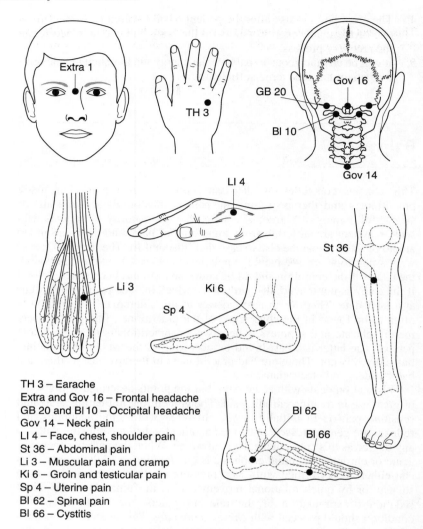

TH 3 – Earache
Extra and Gov 16 – Frontal headache
GB 20 and Bl 10 – Occipital headache
Gov 14 – Neck pain
LI 4 – Face, chest, shoulder pain
St 36 – Abdominal pain
Li 3 – Muscular pain and cramp
Ki 6 – Groin and testicular pain
Sp 4 – Uterine pain
Bl 62 – Spinal pain
Bl 66 – Cystitis

This is a very apt description, because the point is used in 'getting rid of things', i.e. pain, stiffness, negative emotions, sluggishness of the bowel etc. In traditional Chinese medicine (TCM) terms, the point is said to expel wind-heat. It has a remarkable influence on the face and head, so it can help relieve nasal congestion, sneezing, iritis and the symptoms of hay fever. It also helps, in tandem with a powerful lung meridian point (Lu 7 or Lu 9), with sore throats, stiff necks etc. It has an excellent track record in the relief of pain. Either by itself or in conjunction with other points it is used in treating painful syndromes around the face, head, shoulder and abdomen. It is also very useful in treating emotional and mental aggravations, being one of the first points to be tried in the treatment of anxiety (with Li 3), brain fog (with Extra 1) or depression (with St 36). Because this point is so powerful in excretion from the body and mind, it is contra-indicated in the first few months of pregnancy and also during the first 2 days of menstruation. The alternative used on such occasions is LI 11, but even this point should not be stimulated with too much enthusiasm at such times. LI 11, though, has a limited effect on facial and head pain. This aspect of LI 4 can be turned to an advantage, however, during the last few days of pregnancy. It can be used as an excellent distal point in relief of labour pains and also to help in delivery (with Sp 6 and other points).

Li 3

Li 3 is situated at the proximal aspect between the first and second metatarsals. The main action of this point is to subdue liver Yang, and in this, it is frequently used in the treatment of headaches and migraine. It is also the specific point to use in the treatment of cramp. It does not have to be just calf cramp; it can help with cramp in any muscle. It is particularly helpful in abdominal spasms during exercise, i.e. stitch. It also has a profound calming effect on the mind. It is the point of choice to use with patients who are very anxious, frightened or out of sorts. When used in combination with LI 4, the four points are called the four gates, and are often used at the beginning of a treatment session. It is also used in treating hangovers and other excesses of the poor old liver. The mental aspect of liver Yang is anger and frustration. It is used extensively in treating this. The physical counterpart of liver energy is the muscles. It can, therefore, be used in the treatment of generalized muscle soreness, stiffness, spasticity and flaccidity (and the pain that these syndromes entail). Li 3 is said to be the foot equivalent of LI 4. If the hand is placed over the foot, with the thumb being superimposed on the great toe and the little finger on the little toe, it can be seen that the two points are positioned in the same place. This is why the two points are often linked together, because, essentially, they are the same points! This can be done with many other command points. Examples would be GB 41 and TH 3, Sp 6 and P 6, Bl 62 and Si 3 etc.

St 36

This point is one of the most used points in acupressure. It is located one finger's breadth from the anterior crest of the tibia between it and the fibula. It is an extremely versatile point that can be used in pain relief and general energetic conditions. In TCM terms, it is said to tonify Chi and blood where they are deficient. It runs through the whole spectrum of illness, being used in very acute conditions and being also a very useful point in energy depletion and old age. It is used in headaches that have been caused by faulty eating, in cases of gastralgia and abdominal pain, in painful and tired eyes, and in large bowel discomfort. It is one of the best points to use in chronic conditions to boost the body's general energy system. Traditional Chinese medicine would use moxa, but experience has shown that stimulating massage over a period of a few minutes a day is equally effective. Be careful not to stimulate this point too much in cases of gastralgia, nausea and diarrhoea – it could make them all worse.

Sp 4

This point is located on the medial aspect of the foot in a depression at the anterior and inferior border of the first metatarsal bone. It is one of the 'key' points of the eight extraordinary meridians and has such wide-ranging effects on hormonal control, especially of the uterus. It may be used to treat stomach and lower abdominal pain as well as period pain. It is the latter that it has most use in acupressure. It is very useful in the treatment of all uterine pain – menstrual, cervical and even in endometriosis. Although Sp 6 has the honour of being the most versatile point on the spleen meridian, it does not have the anaesthetic qualities of Sp 4.

Ki 6

This point is situated just below the medial malleolus. It is a major point with many functions. It is a good point in the relief of painful areas of the body that also exhibits a certain amount of dryness. It is therefore excellent in the treatment of dry painful eye and throat conditions, also earache where there is some superficial eczema. The point also influences the uterus and can be used in amenorrhoea and uterine prolapse (with Sp 6). It can also be used in chest pain in combination with Ki 27 and P 6. It also represents a useful point in the treatment of testicular and groin pain.

Bl 62

Bl 62 is located just distal to the lateral malleolus, so is positioned directly opposing Ki 6. This point is best known as being an excellent distal point in the treatment of low back pain. It is also useful in the treatment of conjunctivitis, upper cervical and outer leg pain. It is one of the 'key' points of the eight extraordinary meridians with its partner being Si 3. These two points in tandem work well together in spinal pain. They were discussed at length in the last book.

Bl 66

This point is located in the depression anterior and inferior to the fifth metatarso-phalangeal joint. It is a useful point when considering eye pain, headache and stiff neck, but its most useful attribute is in the treatment of acute cystitis, especially in the initial stages of the condition where there is much localized heat and inflammation.

TH 3

This point is located on the posterior aspect of the hand, between the fourth and fifth metacarpals and proximal to the metacarpo-phalangeal joint. This point is not given the recognition that it deserves when described in the various acupuncture tomes. It probably has a more powerful action when used in acupressure. Its influence is three-fold. Firstly, it is used either by itself or in combination with other points (TH 5 and LI 4) in the treatment of earache. Secondly, it is used in the symptomatic relief of hot flushes. Thirdly, it can be a very useful psychosomatic point in the treatment of acute depression and mood swings.

Gov 14

This point is located between the spinous processes of C7 and T1 in the midline. Because of its geography, this point is very useful when used as a local point in the treatment of painful and stiff necks. It is also used in sore throat, shoulder pain and can be of help in the easing of brain fog and dizziness. It is said to be the posterior physical counterpart of the throat chakra and is useful in combination with the anterior point Con 22 in treatment of many conditions that are caused by lack of self-expression. These include depression, constipation, sore throats, chronic fatigue syndrome and painful shoulders.

GB 20 and Bl 10

When it comes to pain relief, these two points are often described together as they have a similar role. GB 20 is located between the origins of the sterno-cleido-mastoid and trapezius muscles at the outer rim of the cranial base. Bl 10 is located 1.5 cun lateral to the midline at the C1–2 level. Together they make a formidable coupling in the treatment of occipital and cranial headache, migraine and brain fog. GB 20 is the more powerful point, and when used in isolation can clear lateral head pain and also headaches caused by overindulgence of fatty foods and alcohol. Bl 10 is useful in the treatment of eyestrain and also as a distal point in the treatment of low back pain.

Extra 1 and Gov 16

The use of these two points will be discussed in Chapter 6.

5

Treatment of chronic conditions

The treatment of chronic conditions is quite different from the treatment of acute ones. Acute conditions represent the 'here and now' in therapeutic care, whereas chronic medical conditions represent the sum of a person's life. When a patient comes for treatment, it has to be understood that whatever the condition being presented, it is there as a result of acute conditions, illnesses, stresses and strains that have been endured for several years. Illnesses do not just happen. Although it is acceptable to manipulate just one point in the case of acute illness, it is not acceptable to do so when treating chronic illness. The treatment of chronic conditions takes time – it has to be worked at, by both therapist and patient. It is unfortunate that many patients consult complementary medicine practitioners as a last resort, after they have done the rounds of doctors and orthodox therapists. Also, because in their eyes, complementary medicine is seen to be 'different', they equate that as being 'instant'. I have despaired, when telling someone with chronic disease that at least half a dozen sessions would be needed, only to be stared at in disbelief. They assumed that it would take one session and some home exercises! It is also important to realize that acupressure and reflextherapy have their limitations, although they are excellent forms of therapy and can work marvels, they do not work every time. A good practitioner knows when to refer the patient to another therapist who may specialize in a form of therapy that is more suitable. As was stated in the previous book, acupressure and reflextherapy may have to be administered to the patient at the same time as them having drug therapy, manipulative therapy etc. Be prepared to mix and match!

Assessment of chronic medical conditions

The assessment is based upon the maxim of look, listen and palpate. It goes without saying that a comprehensive case history is taken – this is now a legal requirement. It has to be legible and written in simple script. The 'look' and 'listen' can be broken down into assessing the patient's constitutional strengths and weaknesses. Once this knowledge is to hand, the treatment programme can be formulated. Most chronic conditions lend themselves towards involvement of a particular organ or system, although this should never be taken for granted. Differentiating a patient's constitutional type is not as difficult as it may seem. There are several ways that can be adopted. The anatomist and kinesiologist would use the body somatyping of mesomorph, ectomorph and endomorph. From this, they would be able to deduce the person's capabilities, strengths and weaknesses. The classically trained homoeopath would use the hereditary weaknesses that show up in the miasms. The Ayurvedic practitioner would archetype using the Ida (deep or organic) and Pingala (superficial and non-organic) strengths and weaknesses. Pure archetypes are rare though and patients exhibit a combination and mixture. A good traditional Chinese medicine (TCM) way of deciding a patient's constitution is by archetyping them through a working knowledge of the law of five elements, as follows:

Water

People have soft features, often dark complexion. They tend to be slow, lazy and adaptable. They would have a tendency to have weak spines and also have kidney, bladder or prostate troubles. They would also have a leaning towards arthritis (especially osteoarthritis) and would be worst in winter and for rest. Patients tend to shuffle. They have extreme fears and phobias amongst the five element types. They dream of drowning and voyages.

Wood

These people have hard, tight and strong musculature. Organized and tense. They have sudden rigid movements. They would have a tendency to weaknesses of the liver and gall bladder. They suffer from headaches, migraines and allergies. They feel symptomatically worse in the spring. They have a tendency to stoop and to have round shoulders. They also speak with a 'drawl' or 'whining' tone that can be very irritating. Emotionally they get angry, irritable and indifferent towards others. They dream of violence.

Fire

Fire people have fine, pointed features, wide foreheads and high cheekbones. Sometimes have ruddy complexions. They tend to be nervous and anxious when giving their history and can also be euphoric and 'giggly'. They also tend to 'gabble' and chatter. They get very anxious and agitated. They tend to suffer from circulatory troubles as well as having cardiac and small bowel imbalances. They dislike extremes in temperature and feel worse in themselves just before lunch and in the middle of the summer. Dream of laughter, being shut in and exposed.

Earth

Earth people have a tendency to be heavy set, often flaccid with a tendency to being overweight. Sallow complexion, if not slightly yellow. Slow moving, calm and practical. They tend to have digestive disorders, also immune system imbalance and also suffer from cold extremities. They do not like wet weather. They have a tendency towards depression and anxiety. Earth people tend not to express themselves readily and can be most frustrating when they insist in not giving the practitioner the whole picture. They dream of food and feasting and that the body is heavy.

Metal

These people are broad-shouldered, but often hollow chested and lean. They have white, pale complexions. They are careful in their movement, enjoying stillness. They are rational people but tend to be melancholic and sad. They dwell on the past. Would have a tendency towards skin and respiratory complaints, also constipation and stiff joints. They feel at their worst in the early morning and late summer. They tend to sit on the front of the chair when talking. They have many fears but not so many as the Water type. They are basically shy and although 'loud' may not express themselves easily. They cry a lot and need to be alone to express grief and sorrow.

The above archetypes should prove to be helpful. They are based purely on traditional teachings. I have used them for many years and find them far more helpful than astrological sun signs or using Chinese astrology.

Having taken a comprehensive case history, watched and listened, the time is right to palpate. This must be done gently and with due care. Please respect the patient's privacy and space. Do not approach them with undue haste. Placing hands on them is also invading their space. They need to be comfortable both physically and mentally with the whole concept of 'hands-on' treatment. Palpation assessment in chronic conditions differs slightly from those used in acute ones. In the following order, this comprises of:

1. Tsing points

Tsing point palpation initially gives the therapist a good idea of the overall energy make up of the patient. Even when there is a relatively normal energy flow in a particular meridian, the Tsing point is slightly tender to the touch. When there is a Yang overtone to the channel, the point is very tender and when the channel is lacking in energy (Yin) the point is almost numb. The points should be stimulated for a few seconds, asking the patient the particular sensation that is being felt.

2. Abdominal alarm points

The sensation felt when massaging these points is different when the corresponding meridian/organ is deficient in energy. It will feel quite dull to the touch, unlike meridians that have adequate Chi, which will feel a little tender (see Figure 2.6).

3. Associated effect points (back transporting point)

The associated effect points (AEP) can prove to be very useful in both assessment and treatment. Please refer to Figure 3.5 for point locations. The points lie on the inner bladder line adjacent to the spine, and are very easy and convenient to palpate. When there is normal sensation of energy flowing through a channel, the AEP will feel 'normal'. If there is a Yin condition and much sluggishness in the meridian, the point will be tender.

This is the reverse of the abdominal points. This, quite often, takes some getting used to, as the therapist is used to dealing with tender points meaning Yang conditions. Another very important consideration is that the inner bladder points mostly equate to the bilateral spinal Chapman's reflexes. It is therefore possible to commence some treatment at the same time as the assessment. Details of how to massage the Chapman's reflexes will be given later in the chapter.

4. Listening post points

These have all been previously described. They are very useful in assessment and subsequent treatment. As has been previously stated, the listening posts are somewhat of an advanced technique. It is important that the rudimentary procedures of acupressure and reflextherapy are known and practised before these methods are used.

So far, the assessment of the condition has used TCM methods and terminology. How does this tie in with Western medical terminology and expression? This is a question that has been asked of me thousands of times, and it is not easy to answer. If the therapist's roots are in traditional medicine (acupressure, reflexology, aromatherapy etc.), they will probably use traditional and naturopathic terminology. If the therapist is trained in Western and allopathic medicine (physiotherapy, chiropractic etc.), they tend to use Western medical terminology. Any orthodox practitioner who has also studied complementary medicine to any degree tends to live a schizophrenic existence. Do they describe chronic asthma as being 'a reversible obstructive lung disorder characterized by increased responsiveness of the airways', or do they describe it as being 'an invasion of wind-cold and an accumulation of damp-phlegm which causes insufficiency of spleen Yang and subsequent lung nourishment'? Oh dear, it is a tricky one! The only advice that can be given to an aspiring acupressure and reflextherapy practitioner is to know which of the main energy channels are affected and how these are translated into the Western concept of named conditions. Western medicine has a tendency to compartmentalize conditions, whereas complementary medicine looks at the person as a whole. This dichotomy and dilemma just has to be overcome, but there is not a simple formula that exists. It just has to be learnt! Subsequently, following the definition of the various named conditions later in the chapter, a traditional diagnosis will also be given.

Principles of treatment

The principles of treatment in chronic conditions are:

1. To ease the presenting symptoms. This could be pain, swelling, dysfunction, stiffness or any other distressing symptom.
2. To improve the Chi energy within the affected organ or system so that the symptoms of the condition do not quickly return.
3. To improve the general level of Chi energy so as to make the patient feel better within.

4.   To instruct home exercises and point stimulation to enable treatment to be continued on a regular basis.

Although all four of the principles are important, it is number 3 that is the most important of all. In good naturopathic tradition, if a patient is made to feel better, that is worth more, to themselves and to the practitioner, than to have superficial symptoms eased. It is far better for the patient to report back after a couple of treatment sessions informing the therapist that they are sleeping better, have more energy and are generally feeling better within than to say that the symptoms have eased but that they themselves feel ill. The latter is bad medicine We have become used to this in allopathic medicine, where the drugs ease the symptoms but create so many ghastly side effects which often create more devastation than the original condition. In acupressure, it is the patient's own vital force that is utilized, not any outside agent. The practitioner merely holds or stimulates the correct acupoint, but essentially it is the patient that heals him or herself without the use of any artificial aid.

The principles of treatment can be achieved by doing the following in the order shown:

1.   Meridian massage of the associated channel(s).
2.   Chapman's reflex massage.
3.   Stimulation of the great point for the condition.
4.   Stimulation and energy balance of the great point with special points.
5.   Stimulation of the energy point for the condition.
6.   Balancing of the body's energy using the Sheng cycle.

1. Meridian massage of the associated channels

The main emphasis in the treatment of most chronic conditions is to stimulate Chi. This is directly opposite to what was done in treating acute conditions. Therefore the meridian massage which is the overture to the session has to concentrate in improving Chi to the underlying energy channels. The channels are stroked between 10 and 12 times in the direction of the energy flow. It can be performed through thin clothing, although where possible, it is better to stroke the skin. Both channels of a bilateral meridian should be stroked, although this is not always a practicality. Make sure that the emphasis of the meridian strokes is made on the areas of the meridians that encompass the command points, i.e. from the fingers to the elbows and between the toes and the knees. This is where the flow of the body's Chi is at its most prolific.

2. Chapman's reflex massage

Here is seen an immediate departure from the routine of treating acute conditions. Chapman's reflexes represent a very underused facet in therapeutic bodywork. It seems that they are not fashionable. Experience, though, has shown that they can be extremely useful in the overall plan of treatment. There are two ways of using them. They can either be massaged as a whole or by just stimulating the ones applicable to the condition. As it only takes a couple of minutes to stimulate all of them, it is preferable to do that. This, though, is a personal preference. There is nothing wrong with massaging just the areas that are applicable – the desired results will still be obtained. Whichever way it is done, it is imperative that the patient is warned beforehand what to expect. Chapman's reflex massage ranks alongside connective tissue massage as being the most painful of all bodywork procedures. They are probably two of the most effective. They have, though, to be performed in context and not abused.

3. Stimulation of the great point for the condition

The word 'great' is not to be used here in context of there being one great point for each meridian. The word 'great' is coined here because it is the only word that can possibly describe the effect that the point has on the treatment of the condition. Quite simply, it is the best and most effective point. The great and special points have all been chosen with the hindsight of 30 years' experience. They do not necessarily represent the points that are most often indicated in acupuncture textbooks. Acupressure is quite different; the points used often have different qualities. The great point is used if there were no other points available. In direct opposition to the treatment of acute conditions, this point *has* to be stimulated. It can be performed with either the finger or thumb pad in a circular movement for up to 5 minutes. This is a long time in which to stimulate a single point, but in chronic conditions, the Chi is so low and deep within the person that it often needs that amount of time to have any effect. If it is possible to stimulate the bilateral points of both left and right meridians, this is more effective and quicker. The therapist's posture often determines whether this is done or not. After about a minute of stimulating the point, some heat will be felt under the finger/thumb pad. The more the massage is done, the more heat will be produced. This is simply heat conduction between two moving objects. After about 2 minutes, a loosening and slackening of the tissues should be felt. This is followed by a generalized warmth and 'oneness' sensation. Do not be surprised if the patient takes a deep breath at this stage of the proceedings – this indicates the movement of Chi and the commencement of relaxation. The point is stimulated until this sensation is felt, although experience is often required as to the exact time. If the thumb pad is used, it must be changed for the finger pad for the remainder of the treatment session, because in the energy balancing that follows, the thumb pad should not be used. Please refer to Figure 1.6 as to which fingers to use.

4. Stimulation and energy balancing of the great point with special points

Each chronic condition has special points that can be used to supplement the great point. Each of the special points has slightly different actions, so not all of them need be used; only those that are pertinent to the patient's symptoms. The special points are derived from local, distal, parallel and vertical zone acupoints plus foot, face and hand reflex points. Each of them has been discovered over a period of time by the author as being the most effective points for a particular condition. It does not mean to say that other points may not be used, each one represents a personal choice. The use of the special points represents the most important and effective part of the whole treatment. The procedure with using each of the special points is as follows:

Stimulate the point for about a minute or two until heat and relaxation of the tissues is felt. Place the same finger of the other hand on the great point and stimulate both points for a further minute following this. Now the points should be held until a balance of energy is felt under the fingers. The balance should be one where a change of emphasis is noted. This occurs when there is brain wave harmony between patient and therapist in the alpha–theta wavelength at 8 c.p.s. This procedure represents the most important part of the whole treatment. As one delegate pointed out – 'it is the difference between curing and just helping'. 'Curing' is the word that he used. I would never use that word in any acupressure procedure: it sets a dangerous precedent. Each of the special points needs to be treated in this manner and this is where the bulk of the treatment time is spent. Less time is needed to balance the points with subsequent treatments because there is more created energy and harmony with each subsequent visit.

5. Stimulation of the energy point for the condition

With using all this energy for healing, what, you may ask, is *the* energy point? One of the principles of treatment was to ease the patient's symptoms sufficiently so that they do not return quickly. This can only be achieved if the specific system and meridian being used in treatment is energized. This is performed by using a powerful point on the 'mother' meridian, based upon the law of five elements. Traditional Chinese medicine says that when a system is weak (Yin), the mother should be fed (in order to feed the son). The point should be stimulated for about 1 minute. During my early years in clinical acupressure, it was not a procedure that I used, but since adopting it, the results have been much better. For those readers who are computer-literate (that is probably all of you), equate this technique with saving the material on disk: it is a back-up system.

6. Balancing of the body's energy using the Sheng cycle

This procedure was also carried out when treating acute conditions to 'finish off' the procedure and to create a good relaxing sensation within the patient. With chronic condition treatment, it is the tonification points of the Yin organs that are used and not the Yang ones. The organ/meridians with their respective points are as follows: spleen (Sp 2) – lung (Lu 11) – kidney (Ki 7) – liver (Li 8) – heart (Ht 7) – pericardium (P 9) (Figure 5.1). When the points are balanced around the Sheng cycle, either the heart or pericardium may be used in the Fire element, not both. Each set of two points used must be stimulated for half a minute prior to a balance being created. It should not be necessary to hold these points for longer than 20 seconds or so. It is only necessary to balance one side of the body.

Treatment of named chronic conditions

The choosing of chronic conditions to treat with acupressure and reflextherapy was not an easy task. Delegates and students who knew this book was being written made the decision from a consensus of opinion. It had to consist of conditions that are treated on an everyday basis by both orthodox and complementary practitioners. Musculo-skeletal conditions had already been covered in the first book and acute conditions had also been discussed in the previous chapter. There are probably, though, many

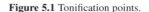

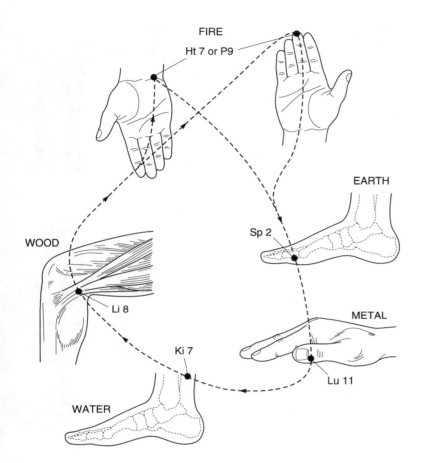

Figure 5.1 Tonification points.

conditions that have not been mentioned that ideally lend themselves to treatment by bodywork techniques. The discerning reader and therapist will, though, be able to formulate the treatment of most conditions from the templates that are given in the undermentioned named conditions.

Chronic bronchial asthma

Definition: A reversible obstructive lung disorder characterized by increased responsiveness of the airways.

The lungs are the organs responsible for the transformation and distribution of Chi and regard asthma as a series of symptoms associated with a variety of perverse influences on lung function. These may come from an inherent factor or from external causes such as allergic reactions, infection and stress. There is usually coughing, shortness of breath and stringy sputum that is difficult to expectorate due to bronchiole spasm. Orthodox treatment is normally by broncho-dilatory drugs and breathing exercises.

Figure 5.2 Points used in chronic asthma.

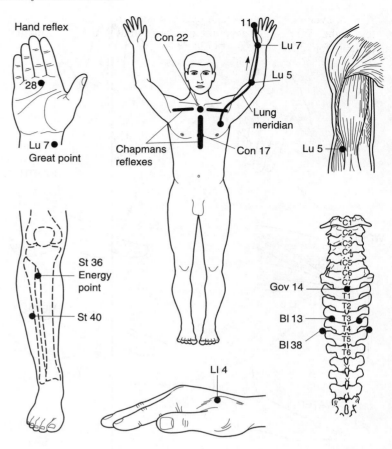

Acupressure and reflextherapy treatment (see Figure 5.2)

1. The associated meridian is the lung channel. This should be stroked at least 10 times in the direction of energy flow, i.e. from the chest towards the thumb. This can easily be performed bilaterally with the patient in either lying or long sitting.
2. The associated Chapman's reflexes are to be found under the clavicles and down the sternum. These areas are to be massaged, using two or three finger pads together, with some degree of strength. As has been stated before, it is essential that the patient be warned that the massage will be painful.
3. The great point in the condition is Lu 7. It is located on the radial side of the forearm, 1.5 cun proximal to the transverse wrist crease. It is one of *the* great points in acupuncture and acupressure and is used to treat many respiratory conditions. It is said to be the 'oxygen' point of the lungs, as it tends to ease broncho-spasms and enable the patient to expectorate more easily. The point should be stimulated bilaterally for about 5 minutes. This should be done in a slow rhythmical manner. This kind of stimulation is a halfway house between boring a hole in the patient's tissues and polishing the skin. It has to be effective without being painful or ineffectual. After 5 minutes of stimulation, the point should feel much warmer and 'harmonious'. The patient

should, even at this early stage of the session, feel that the lungs feel less tight. This is the acupoint of choice that should be taught to patients for self-treatment.

4. There are 10 special points used in this condition. Each one has a slightly different mode of action. There are two more points on the lung meridian, three points over the spine, two points on the sternum, two distal points and a hand reflex point for patient use. Lu 1 and Lu 5 may be used to ease broncho-spasm and ease breathing. Do not press on Lu 1 too much; it is a very tender point and has to be treated with respect. Lu 1 is also a good point to relieve coughing. Lu 5 is useful where there is much phlegm. Bl 13 and Bl 38 are used in tandem. Bl 13 is located over the transverse process between T3 and T4, whilst Bl 38 lies on the 'outer bladder' line between T4 and T5. Bl 13 is the back transporting point of the lungs, and as such is used to stimulate energy in the lungs. It should also be stimulated when there is much heat in the system, scanty sputum and a red tongue. Bl 38 may be added when there are stress overtones to the condition. St 40 is located halfway down the lateral aspect of the lower leg, 8 cun below the knee joint. It is a very useful distal point when there is much copious phlegm. It has the effect of opening the chest and easing breathing. It is also a very good point in anxiety and tension, which often overrides this condition. It can also be used in pain relief around the throat and upper chest. The better pain relief point, however, is LI 4. This is very useful in treating the soreness of the chest and ribs that accompanies constant coughing. It can also serve to relax the chest. Do not stimulate this point if the patient is pregnant. Hand reflex 28 is a useful point taught to the patient to ease tension in the chest. They should be encouraged to stimulate this point and Lu 7 each hour during the day for about 2 or 3 minutes. The final special points have an influence on relieving the stress that accompanies (or causes) this condition. Con 22 coupled with Gov 14 will be mentioned in the next chapter. Con 17 will also be mentioned in Chapter 6 as being a superb point in anxiety and distress, but it can also be used to wonderful effect in asthma. It dispels fullness from the chest and aids breathing. When balancing the many special points with Lu 7, it will be found that the distal and spinal points take longer to energy balance than do the sternal points. As mentioned before, it is not necessary to use all the points, just the salient ones. The most important thing to remember when balancing Lu 7 with each special point is that this part of the treatment represents the most important facet part. It is essential in order to have any effect in the course of the disease that a change of emphasis is made.

5. The associated 'energy' point is St 36. Not only is this point probably the best point in the body for improving general energy, but it happens to be the great point of the Earth element, which is the mother of the Metal element, the lung meridian being the Yin component.

6. It is now time to give a final energy balance via the tonification points of the Yin channels via the Sheng cycle. The therapist may start anywhere on the 'circle' provided that the circle is completed.

Non-acupressure treatment

It is always a good thing if the acupressure and reflextherapy treatment of any condition can be supplemented with input from other disciplines and philosophies, providing that there is no conflict that may cause the patient discomfort. I have always been a strong advocate of thinking holistically about treatment and have never been afraid to suggest other forms of approach where the need arises. Acupressure does not necessarily suit everyone, nor is it always the ideal therapy. In the case of chronic asthma, the obvious treatment that comes to mind is to make sure that the thoracic spine, sternum, posterior rib facet joints and costal joints are gently mobilized. This can be achieved with Maitland mobilization or with any of the gentler approaches of osteopathy or McTimony chiropractic. It is hopeless to just treat the patient with subtle energy techniques if the underlying joints and soft tissues need adjustment or mobilizing. As any osteopath or chiropractor will know, the movement of the underlying structure provides its own kind of energy release. It is also obvious to the practitioner that if the patient is suffering from allergic reactions, that the allergies are ascertained by one of a number of methods that are available. Ensure that the patient's food intake is natural and wholesome and that all preservatives, additives and refined carbohydrates are avoided. This condition is also the ideal one for constitutional homoeopathic prescribing. Make sure that the homoeopath is qualified and experienced.

Chronic obstructive pulmonary disease (COPD)

Definition: Generalized airways obstruction, particularly of small airways, associated with varying combinations of chronic bronchitis, asthma and emphysema.

It is often very difficult for physicians to diagnose the difference between chronic bronchitis, asthma and emphysema. They are therefore placed together under the umbrella term of COPD. The treatment for this group of conditions obviously includes points used in the treatment of asthma, as it forms part of the triad, but the reader will ascertain several differences in the treatment of COPD.

Acupressure and reflextherapy treatment (see Figure 5.3)

1. The associated meridians in COPD are the lung and spleen channels. These should be stroked about 10 times each in the direction of energy movement. It is best to stroke the spleen meridian first to the lateral aspect of the chest, then proceed to the lung channel in one continuous movement.
2. The relevant Chapman's reflexes are the same as those in asthma, namely along the underside of the clavicles and down the sternum. Remember the warning given to patients!
3. The great point for this combination is Lu 9. This point is located at the lateral side of the anterior wrist crease. It is the source point of the lungs; therefore it has direct energy access to the lungs. It is the best point on the lung channel to use in chronic obstructive conditions. It is

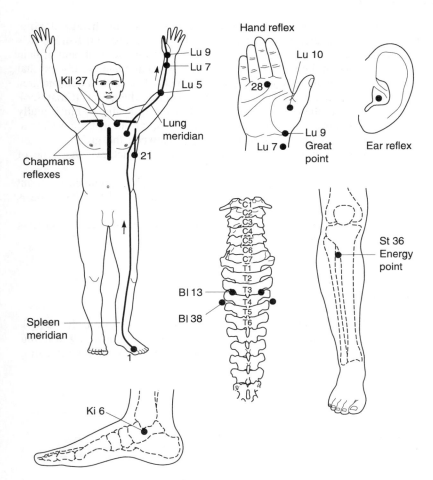

Figure 5.3 Points used in chronic obstructive pulmonary disease.

useful in tonifying energy, resolving phlegm and easing out sticky chests. The point (or bilateral points) should be given stimulating massage for about 5 minutes or until such time as a definite change of feeling is noted in the tissues around the point.

4. There are 10 special points. Four are located on the lung meridian, one on the chest, two on the spine, one distal point at the ankle, and there are reflex points on the hand and ear. The actions of Lu 1, Lu 5 and Lu 7 have previously been mentioned. Lu 10 is located on the mound of the thumb. If a pin is placed straight through the flesh at LI 4, it will emerge at Lu 10. This point is the Fire point of the lung meridian and is used when there is heat and fullness obstructing the chest (as in bronchitis). It can also be used in the treatment of sore throats. Ki 27 is the last point on the kidney meridian, located inferior to the medial end of the clavicle. It is used similarly to Lu 1 as a local point. Use it especially when the patient is very tired and low in energy, also when they may be having difficulty in urinating due to cortisone drugs. The distal point of Ki 6 is located at the distal end of the medial malleolus. It is of especial use when there is dryness in the chest or when there is great difficulty in expectorating. It is an important point used in the treatment of any condition of the elderly. Bl 13 and Bl 38 have been

previously described in the last condition, as has the hand reflex no. 28. There is also a special point in the ear (would you believe it is called the lung point). This point is very good in the treatment of pain and is one of the four points (with Lu 7, Lu 9 and hand reflex 28) that can be given to patients for home treatment. The ear is a delicate area and great care must be taken when massaging this point. It may look odd to poke the ear with a baby bud or the little finger, but it really works. On the topic of hand and ear reflexes, it is almost impossible to achieve a change of emphasis balance between the great point and these reflex points. The best reflected area to achieve this type of balance is the foot.

5. The energy point is once again St 36. It should be stimulated for about 2 minutes. At subsequent sessions, it will be found that less time is needed to effectively treat this point.
6. Now balance the body's general energy using the tonification points on the Sheng cycle.

Non-acupressure treatment

Please refer to the advice given with the previous condition, the same is pertinent. Insist that the patient also increase their fitness by walking, swimming or cycling. This is an excellent way of improving lung function.

Chronic rhinitis and sinusitis

Definition: Rhinitis is an upper respiratory infection, characterized by oedema and vasodilatation of the nasal mucous membrane, nasal discharge and obstruction. Sinusitis is an inflammatory process in the paranasal sinuses due to viral, bacterial or fungal infections or local allergic reactions.

The pain and discomfort suffered in rhinitis and sinusitis has been likened to boiling a can of beans with the lid still secured. The treatment of the acute counterpart of this condition was discussed in the last chapter. The chronic version of this condition has worse pain and discomfort. As well as the above causes, sinusitis often occurs due to the person being 'stuck' in a groove and unhappy with their lot. Because it is a condition that involves the excretory system of the body, skin conditions and constipation often accompany it.

Acupressure and reflextherapy treatment (Figure 5.4)

1. The associated meridians in these conditions are the lung and large intestine channels. These should be stroked 10 times in the direction of energy flow.
2. The Chapman's reflexes are situated under the clavicles, down the

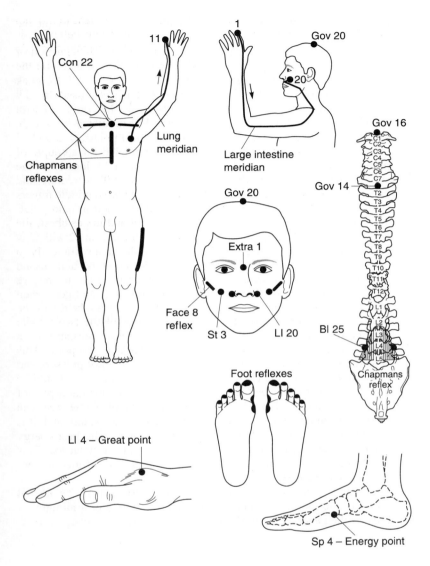

Figure 5.4 Points used in chronic rhinitis and sinusitis.

sternum, down the ileo-tibial tracts on the lateral aspect of the upper legs and a large triangular area above the sacrum. All these areas are very sore and the patient must be informed that they may 'hover' above the couch for the duration of the massage. It is especially true of the ileo-tibial tract. This area is commonly massaged in the treatment of low back pain, colitis, constipation and coldness of the limbs. It should be massaged with oil. To make it even more effective, try to do some connective tissue massage down this line.

3. The great point for these two conditions is LI 4. It is the ideal point because it combines its action of pain relief and congestion relief as well as stimulating the excretory organ of the large intestine. LI 4 should be massaged bilaterally for about 5 minutes. It is also an ideal point to be used by the patient at home. Do *not* use this point when the patient is pregnant or in the first 2 days of menstruation. The

alternative points are either LI 11 (at the elbow) or LI 15 (at the shoulder).

4. There are 10 special points that can be used to reinforce the action of LI 4, each having a slightly different action. Bl 25 is situated on the inner bladder between the transverse processes of L4–L5. It is the back transporting point of the large intestine and can be used in any excretory sluggishness. This point can, obviously, be combined with the Chapman's reflex in the area. It should be stimulated in chronic and long-standing conditions. There are two local points, St 3 and LI 20. Both of these points should be gently stimulated for a couple of minutes before balancing with LI 4. Face reflex area 8 is located on the side of the face underneath the zygomatic arch. When treating and energy balancing, a wide spread positioning of the three middle fingers should be employed. This balance is particularly good in pain relief. Together with other conditions around the head and upper chest, the two-point energy balance of Extra 1 with Gov 16 and Con 22 with Gov 14 has proved to be very effective in relaxing the area sufficiently to allow easier passage of mucus. Gov 20, the point of a thousand meetings (crown chakra), is an excellent point used to relieve congestion in the head. The technique is a simple one and performed with the patient in supine lying. Place both hands across the top of the head with the fingers spread a little and the tips of the two middle fingers opposing each other. Gradually increase pressure in a downward and outwards movement, so as to 'stretch' the point. This is held for up to 5 minutes. It can give enormous relief of pressure and discomfort. Finally, the classical points of the foot reflexes should be used. These points lie on the tips of the toes, on the medial aspect of the great toe and medial aspect of the ball of the foot. These areas can be supplemented with the lung and large intestine areas, although it is not necessary to energy balance with these points. The best energy balance point on the foot is the medial aspect of the great toe. This should be balanced with LI 4 for up to 5 minutes. It affords tremendous pain and congestion relief.

5. The energy point for this condition is Sp 4, located on the medial aspect of the foot. It should be stimulated for about 3 or 4 minutes.

6. Finally, the general energy should be balanced via the Sheng cycle.

Non-acupressure treatment

The patient should be encouraged to use lots of garlic in food. Garlic is the most powerful natural cleanser and 'antibiotic' that we have. A useful way of using garlic is to snip a garlic capsule with scissors, allowing the liquid garlic to come out. Place this liquid on the inside of the nostrils and sniff back several times. The downside of this is that friends are few and far between during the procedure. Another natural way of washing out the sinuses is to buy a cheap plastic atomizer and fill it with extremely dilute salt solution (no more than 5 grains of salt per 50 mils of warm water). When squirted up the nostrils, it produces a very fine spray of dilute brine. This should be done twice per day. When the sinuses are very painful, the patient should try homoeopathic Kali Bich 30 throughout the day. Similarly, when very infected they should try Hepar Sulph 30 or colloidal silver on a regular basis.

Impotence

Definition: The inability to attain or sustain an erection satisfactory for normal coitus. The causes are variable – these include chronic anxiety syndrome, hormonal imbalance and a chronic low back condition. There are many more possibilities, but these three were purposely presented to the reader to represent the possible aetiology of this and many other chronic conditions, namely mental (or emotional), chemical and physical. This triad of healing may be represented in most chronic conditions. By using acupressure and reflextherapy, all three possible causes can be addressed – that is the great beauty of bodywork.

Acupressure and reflextherapy treatment (Figure 5.5)

1. The associated meridian in this condition is the kidney channel. This is because the kidney channel represents ancestral energy, is specific in conditions with the kidneys and testes, passes through the region and is excellent in the treatment of many emotional illnesses. It should be bilaterally stroked up to a dozen times in the direction of energy flow from the sole of the foot towards the chest.
2. The Chapman's reflex areas associated with the kidney channel are to be found just inferior to the deltoid insertion on the arm, just superior and lateral to the umbilicus and the wide triangular area above the sacrum. These areas should be stimulated. However, in such a chronic imbalance as this condition, it is much more worthwhile to massage all the reflexes.
3. The great point is Ki 3. This point is located midway between the tip of the medial malleolus and the Achilles tendon. It is the source point of the kidney. When stimulated, it tonifies kidney Chi and generally improves the energy levels around the pelvic region. This point should be stimulated bilaterally for up to 5 minutes. This is also the ideal point that the patient can use at home.
4. There are five special acupoints and reflex areas that can be used in this condition. The most important area by far to treat, is the lower lumbar and sacral region. Bl 23 and Bl 47, located between L2 and L3 are stimulated to help the production of adrenaline and cortisol. The sacral 'bladder' points should be stimulated for about 1 minute each, as well as massaging the whole area. Connective tissue massage coupled with lumbo-sacral soft tissue stretching can also be added at this time. Time should be taken over this procedure – it is very important. It is also a good idea to energy balance Bl 23 with Ki 3 whilst working on the lower spine area. The frontal points of Con 6 and Con 4 are very useful in the treatment of impotence and for strengthening the reproductive system as a whole. An excellent balance may be obtained with Con 6 and Ki 3. The foot reflexes may be used with great effect in this condition. The best areas are those reflected with the bladder, ureter and kidney, plus the ones on the medial and lateral aspects of the heels that are associated with the testes. The large area on the medial aspect of the heel is particularly effective.

Figure 5.5 Points used in impotence.

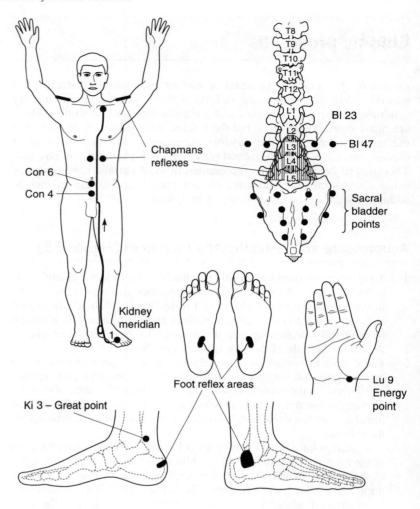

5. The energy point is Lu 9, which is located on the antero-lateral aspect of the wrist. The lung channel is the 'mother' of the kidney.
6. Finally, a general energy balance using the Yin organs of the Sheng cycle should be carried out.

Non-acupressure treatment

As has already been stated, it is vital to improve the movement, hence function, of the lower spine, especially the sacrum. All this can be done at the same time the acupressure is being given. Also teach the patient some back-strengthening exercises. Diet is especially important in this condition. Cut out all refined sugar and eat as many legumes and beans as possible. Pumpkin seeds are also advantageous.

Chronic prostatitis

Definition: A chronic inflammation of the prostate gland caused by bacterial infection or unknown factors. With this condition, the prostate gland swells and can occlude the urethra and seminal vessels. It can be very painful and disabling.

Acupressure and reflextherapy treatment (Figure 5.5)

The procedure for prostatitis is virtually the same as for impotence; although do not get the idea that the two conditions are either related or run concurrently. Personal observation of treating these two conditions, however, supports the idea that one often does lead to the other. The only one of the points used in impotence that should not be used in this treatment is Con 6. All the others are valid.

Dysmenorrhoea

Definition: Cyclical pain associated with menses during ovulatory cycles, but without demonstrable lesions affecting the reproductive cycle. The pain is thought to result from uterine contractions and ischaemia. It is common in adolescent women and tends to decrease with age and following pregnancy, although it can affect older women who may have had no previous trouble. The cause may be a combination of hormonal, structural or emotional factors and acupressure and reflextherapy are ideally suited to treat all these.

Treatment with acupressure and reflextherapy (Figure 5.6)

1. The associated meridians are the kidney and spleen channels. These bilateral channels should be stroked up to 10 times in the flow of energy, i.e. from the feet towards the chest.
2. The Chapman's reflexes are located at the insertion of the deltoid on the side of the arm, two points superior and lateral to the umbilicus, the left costal margin and the area above the sacrum. These areas should be stimulated. Be sure to warn the patient.
3. The great point is Sp 6. This point is located 3 cun superior to the medial malleolus and just posterior to the tibial border. It is a highly influential point in all gynaecological conditions. It is said to be the meeting point of the three Yin channels on the leg (liver, kidney and spleen) and hence influences all three channels. It is useful in all pain cases around the pelvis. It has a marvellous action in 'smoothing out' obstructions and relieving pain. The point should be stimulated for up

Figure 5.6 Points used in dysmennhoria and pelvic inflammatory disease.

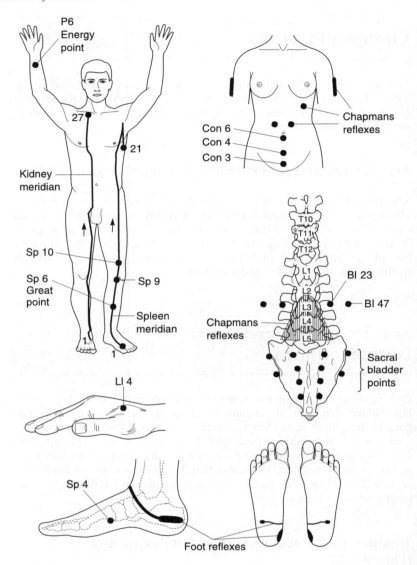

to 5 minutes. It will take less time in the younger woman who has not experienced symptoms for that long.

4.   There are seven special points that can be used in assisting Sp 6 in its action. Three of the points lie on the spleen channel (Sp 4, Sp 9 and Sp 10); two lie on the lower conception channel (Con 4 and Con 6) and two on the spine (Bl 23 and Bl 47). Sp 4 is useful in most gynaecological conditions in that it calms spasm in the uterus and helps regulate menstruation by stopping excessive bleeding. This point should be stimulated for 2 minutes before being energy balanced with Sp 6. Sp 9, located in a depression just below the medial condyle of the tibia, helps to reduce uterine inflammation and 'hot flushes'. In these cases, it should be stimulated for a minute prior to energy balancing with Sp 6. Sp 10 is located in the highest part of the vastus medialis muscle. The point is used in stasis of blood, especially in the

uterus. It is therefore indicated in this condition where there is much clotting and painful periods. It should be stimulated for 2 minutes. The two local points of Con 4 and Con 6 are very useful. Con 4 nourishes blood, hence having an effect on the uterus and menstruation. It also tonifies the kidney channel, thus giving energy to the pelvic area. The balance between Con 4 and Sp 6 is probably the most important one of all the sets of points. Con 6 is said to be the anterior physical component of the sacral chakra and as such is a splendid point to use in cases of swelling, stress and hormonal imbalance. It is used in a plethora of symptoms that include urinary difficulties, vaginal discharge, loose stools, profuse pale urination, physical weakness, mental depression, lack of willpower and 'tired all the time' syndrome. It is a very useful point. This should be balanced with Sp 6 until a change of emphasis is noted. The two points around L2–L3, namely Bl 23 and Bl 47 have been previously described as useful in giving energy to the pelvic area and balancing the adrenal hormones.

5. The energy point is P 6. This is also a master point in the treatment of nausea. Care must be taken not to over-stimulate this point as it could cause sickness.
6. Now balance the general energy via the Sheng cycle.

Non-acupressure treatment

There are many herbal and homoeopathic remedies that can be recommended for this condition. Vitamin B6 and oil of evening primrose are excellent. For cramping, homoeopathic Mag. Phos. 6/30 should be taken every half-hour until it appears easier.

Pelvic inflammatory disease (PID)

Definition: Pelvic inflammatory disease is a term used to include salpingitis (inflammation of the fallopian tubes), cervicitis (inflammation of the cervix), endometriosis (inflammation of the uterus and the presence of endometrial tissue in abnormal places), vaginitis (inflammation of the vagina) and oophoritis (inflammation of the ovaries). In each and every example of inflammation, bacterial infection is normally present. These conditions may occur at any age but are more common at the time of menopause.

Treatment with acupressure and reflextherapy (Figure 5.6)

1. The associated meridians are the kidney and spleen, the same as the last condition. They should be stroked with the flow of energy about 10 times.
2. The Chapman's reflex areas are the same as in dysmenorrhoea.
3. The great point is the same, namely Sp 6. This should be stimulated

bilaterally for up to 5 minutes. This is often enough to help with any degree of pain existing in the pelvic region.

4. There are 11 special points and reflected areas that can be used to supplement the action of Sp 6. In addition to the points described in the previous condition, there are Con 3, the sacral bladder points, the foot reflex areas and the distal pain relief point of LI 4. Con 3 is used primarily in the treatment of cystitis, but is of great use when there is local pain in the uterus, vagina and cervix. Be careful when using this point where there is a lot of discomfort. The stimulation should be gentle and rhythmical. The sacral bladder points are especially useful when there is much congestion and stiffness in the area. These can be massaged at the same time that the Chapman's reflexes are stimulated. The distal pain relief point LI 4 represents a time-honoured combination (with Sp 6) in all pelvic pain. This combination is particularly useful during confinement. It should not, however, be used in the first 8 months of pregnancy or during menstruation. LI 4 in isolation should not be used at any time during pregnancy (except during confinement – see next section). These two points should be taught to a member of the patient's family in order that treatment may be continued at home. The foot reflex areas of the uterus, pelvis and fallopian tubes are excellent when treating these conditions.
5. The energy point is P 6.
6. Balance the general energy via the Sheng cycle.

Obstetrics

Treatment with accupressure and reflextherapy (Figure 5.7)

It is very rewarding to be able to use acupressure and reflextherapy in pregnancy and to be able to deal with any problems that may arise by using gentle, natural and safe methods. In this section, it is not necessary to indicate a great point or energy point because of the individuality of each imbalance. There is, however, an associated meridian in the majority of obstetric imbalances – the spleen. It would be good, therefore, to stroke this channel in the direction of energy in every condition that is encountered. The spleen channel does not have a monopoly though, other meridians are important. These are the kidney, conception and liver.

Infertility

There are many causes of infertility. Acupressure and reflextherapy treatments represent only a small part of the equation in the whole combined effort of attempting to produce fertility. The two points that are recommended that should be used in treatment rooms and by the patient in her own home are Con 6 and Ki 3. Con 6 is a powerful point. It is the physical equivalent of the anterior sacral chakra and is commonly known as the Hara. It is therefore used in general relaxation of the tissues, especially the pelvic region. It is also useful in extreme physical and

Figure 5.7 Points used in obstetrics.

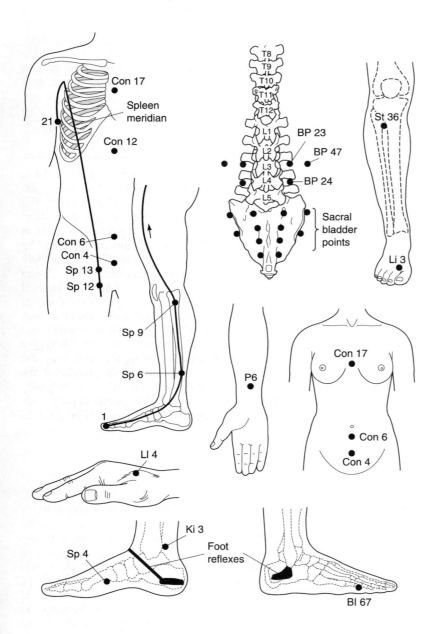

mental exhaustion and depression, which often accompanies infertility. Ki 3 tonifies the kidneys and hence generally improves the ancestral energy. It is also used in the treatment of low back pain, pelvic tension and swollen ankles. These two points should be stimulated for about 5 minutes each every day.

Morning sickness

Three points are indicated. The best one to use is P 6, located 2 cun superior to the anterior wrist crease. It is particularly indicated when there is vomiting as well as nausea. St 36 is the usual point for nausea in non-obstetric conditions, and works very well in early pregnancy sickness. Do not over-stimulate this point just after eating as it can cause vomiting. A good local point to use is Con 12. This can be used in combination with either P 6 or St 36.

Pregnancy discomfort

The only points of contra-indication in the duration of pregnancy are LI 4, Sp 6 and Ki 3. The most common form of discomfort is low back pain. This may be treated with the local points of Bl 23, Bl 47 and Bl 24. The sacral bladder points may also be used in cases where the discomfort envelops the whole of the pelvis. Sp 9 may be used as a distal point in relieving abdominal pain, combined with the local points of Sp 12 and Sp 13. Local and distal acupressure can be done using these points where there is pain and the horrible sensation of lower abdominal distension. Li 3 may be used when the sensation feels more like cramp. Con 4 may also be used as a local point with either Sp 9 or Li 3 in decreasing lower abdominal pain. The foot reflexes that relate to the uterus and fallopian tubes may also be massaged to try and decrease tension and fullness. Sp 4 is another distal point used for pain relief. This point may also be balanced with P 6 to give an all-round relaxation. If there is any anxiety during the pregnancy, the best point to use is Con 17. This point is located in the middle of the sternum and is quite tender when it requires treatment. It should be gently stimulated until the anxiety passes. Other anti-anxiety points in pregnancy are Li 3 and Ki 3. A complete list in generalized anxiety will be given in Chapter 6.

Labour pain

The following points may be used during the very final moments of pregnancy, should the need arise. If the delivery is in a hospital or special unit, always obtain permission of the senior physician or midwife before commencing to use any acupressure. Firstly, it is common courtesy, and secondly it serves to acquaint the staff with the more 'alternative' and natural methods. It goes without saying that permission should also be obtained from the patient. She may have been a long-term client or she may have called for acupressure in the delivery room as an alternative to drugs. Whatever the situation, confidence of the patient and staff must be gained by your procedures. There are three points used in labour analgesia – LI 4, Sp 6 and Li 3. This is the only time that LI 4 and Sp 6 may be used in pregnancy. Remember how LI 4 was described in an earlier chapter – the 'great eliminator'? Here it is used for that very purpose. Care must be taken not to be in too much of a hurry, and also not to get in the way of everyone else in the room. Start by gently massaging LI 4 bilaterally for about 2 minutes. This is followed by massaging Sp 6 bilaterally for about 3 minutes, then Li 3 for a further 2 minutes. This procedure should have relaxed the pelvic region sufficiently that more in-depth stimulation can take place. Position yourself at the patient's side and stimulate LI 4 and Sp 6 at the same time, using the same rhythmical massage. This should produce the desired results.

Breech presentation

Should this occur, Bl 67 may be used to resolve the situation. This point is used extensively in China for turning a breech delivery into normal engagement. The point is mostly given moxa, but acupressure is used extensively. This point is very tender and should be massaged bilaterally using rhythmical stimulation. The courtesy and legal procedures laid down in the previous section are also pertinent in these cases.

Postpartum

Exhaustion is probably the most common 'complication'. St 36 massage is useful, combined with Bl 23 and Bl 47. The latter is particularly effective if there is also some residual backache. Li 3 should be used for headaches and cramps. It is usually the case though, that the mother is so tired and elated that all she wants to do is be alone with the baby and rest as much as possible.

Stress incontinence and enuresis

Definition: The involuntary loss of urine on coughing, straining, sneezing, lifting or movement that increases the intra-abdominal pressure. Enuresis or bed-wetting is the involuntary loss of urine during periods of sleep. Stress incontinence is more common in the elderly and following surgery to the pelvic region. Enuresis is common in all ages. Infantile enuresis often has psychosomatic overtones. The cause of stress incontinence is usually pelvic floor musculature weakness. It may also be present in uterine prolapse.

    The aim of treatment is to strengthen these muscles. Often it is the case that acupressure treatment is only effective in the early stages, when surgery must be considered.

Treatment by acupressure and reflextherapy (Figure 5.8)

1. The associated meridians are the kidney and bladder channels. In all cases, these should be stroked in the direction of energy up to a dozen times for each channel.
2. The Chapman's reflex area to be massaged is the broad triangular area that extends above the sacrum towards L 2/3. At the same time, it would be pertinent to massage the sacral bladder points. Massaging this area relieves congestion and helps to clear the lymphatic channels that may be sluggish.
3. The great point is Bl 62. This point is located just inferior to the lateral malleolus. This point is mostly used as a distal point in the treatment of low back pain. It is its use in acupressure, as opposed to acupuncture, that really shows its versatility. It is used to relax the pelvic region and to strengthen the perineum. Please do not equate

Figure 5.8 Points used in stress incontinence and enuresis.

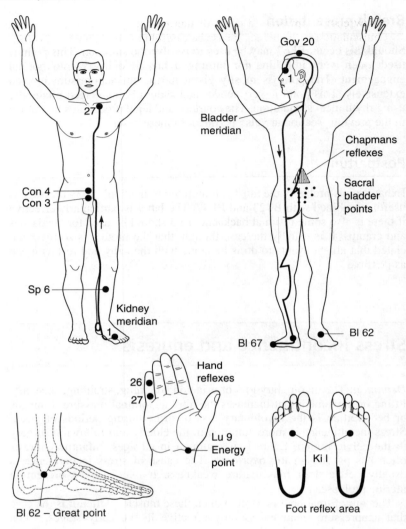

relaxation of muscles to being weak muscles. Muscular spasm equates to weakness; therefore if the spasm can be reduced, the way is open to strengthen the muscles. Following the acupressure treatment, therefore, it is essential that pelvic floor exercises be taught. Bl 62 should be stimulated bilaterally for about 5 minutes.

4.   There are eight special points and reflex areas used to supplement the action of Bl 62. Firstly massage the local points Con 3 and Con 4 for about 3 minutes each. Balancing each point with Bl 62 until a change of emphasis is felt follows this. This action starts to ease the tension in the area of the bladder and perineum. Next, stimulating Sp 6 strengthens the pelvic area. Massage this point for at least 4 minutes before attempting a balance of energy between it and Bl 62. The patient in home treatment may use the two hand reflex points 26 and 27. The broad band foot reflex around the heel is an excellent area to use in cases of pelvic congestion. Finally, a recognized ploy in TCM is to stimulate the 'point of a thousand meetings' at Gov 20 in order to

draw energy upwards in cases of uterine collapse and general weak musculature in the pelvis. Please be careful in stimulating this point as it could cause dizziness and light-headedness. Instead of balancing Gov 20 to Bl 62, the better point for a balance would be Ki 1 on the sole of the foot. In practical terms, this has to be carried out with the patient in the sitting position with the knees bent up (unless the therapist has extremely long arms).

5. The energy point for this condition is Lu 9, located on the lateral aspect of the anterior wrist crease.
6. Finally, balance the general energy via the Sheng cycle.

This treatment has not included the possible psychosomatic causes of enuresis. This will be covered in the next chapter.

Poor circulation (cold hands and feet)

Although this is not a named condition as such, these symptoms can be among the most prominent and uncomfortable of all. There is a multitude of possible causes, and acupressure cannot hope to cater for all of these, but it remains extremely effective in very many cases.

Treatment by acupressure and reflextherapy (Figure 5.9)

1. There are three associated meridians: the liver, pericardium and the three heater. All three should be stroked in the direction of energy flow about eight times each, regardless of which limb has poor circulation.
2. The Chapman's reflexes are situated down the lateral aspect of the upper leg and underneath the costal insertion of the right pectoralis major muscles in the sixth intercostal space. These areas should be massaged with the usual enthusiasm associated with these points.
3. There is not a great point because the cause of each symptom may differ. The special points used are as follows: hand and arm – Con 22, Gov 14, TH 15, LI 15, LI 11 and LI 10; foot and leg – Con 6, Gov 4, Gov 3, St 30, Li 8 and St 36. In addition, there are two hand reflex points, 22 and 23. The aim of the treatment is to stimulate each associated point for about 1 minute, until heat and relaxation is produced. This is commenced at the most proximal point of the limb, progressing downwards. The points chosen are those, with experience in their use, that offers the best solution. *Hand coldness* – Massage both Con 22 and Gov 14 at the same time. These two points represent the anterior and posterior aspects of the throat chakra. After stimulating these two points for about a minute, the lower neck and shoulders should be feeling more relaxed. Next stimulate TH 15. This point is located on the posterior aspect of the trapezius muscle, halfway between the tip of the shoulder and the spine. When this point is stimulated, it improves the circulation to the arm and shoulder. This is followed by stimulating points on the large intestine meridian – LI 15, 11 and 10 – in that order. LI 10 is not a well-known point in acupuncture, but it is a highly effective point in acupressure to

Figure 5.9 Points used in poor circulation.

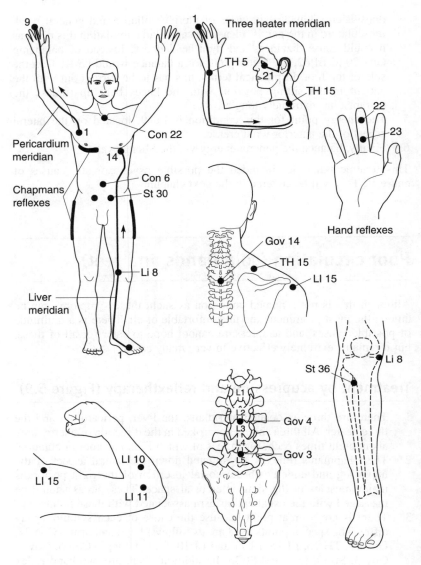

improve the blood and lymphatic circulation to the hand. It is located 2 cun inferior to LI 11. After this point has been massaged, the whole arm should be tingling and feeling much warmer. *Foot coldness* – Start the procedure by giving stimulating massage to both Con 6 and Gov 4 at the same time for about 1 minute. These two points are the physical counterpart of the sacral chakra and are ideally suited for this role. Next stimulate St 30 and Gov 3 simultaneously. Be careful when massaging St 30: it is located in the groin area. Next stimulate Li 8 for a minute, followed by St 36. After a total of 4 minutes, the leg should feel much warmer. Several treatments will be required to give a long-lasting effect.

4. Balance the general body energy via the Sheng cycle.

The two hand reflexes 22 and 23 are located on the anterior aspect of the middle fingers. Patients should be encouraged to massage these at home. Of the other points that are easily accessible in self-healing, LI 10 for the upper limb and Li 8 for the lower limb are the most effective. The patient should be encouraged to massage these two points at least three times a day for a couple of minutes each.

Oedema and water retention

Oedema around the ankles and general water retention may be caused by a number of factors. The simplest causes are mechanical ones – wearing tight fitting shoes, sitting too long (e.g. long plane journey), standing too long (e.g. shop assistant) and being overweight. Other causes are having a salt-rich diet, hormonal imbalance or suffering from cardiac imbalance. Whatever the cause, the undermentioned acupressure techniques will give much relief from the symptoms. In TCM terms, there is always sluggishness with the kidney meridian and sometimes the spleen channel if the cause is hormonal.

Treatment by acupressure and reflextherapy (Figure 5.10)

1. The associated meridians are the kidney, pericardium and lung channels. All three should be stroked in the direction of energy flow about 10 times each. If there is much ankle swelling, emphasize the kidney stroke around the ankle.
2. The Chapman's reflex best suited to this condition is the area down the lateral aspect of the thigh. When there is generalized water retention and cellulite formation, this area is extremely painful. The patient must be warned of this and be tactfully informed that it is doing them the world of good!
3. The great point is Con 6. This point has been discussed before as being the physical counterpart of the sacral chakra, hence having an influence in water imbalance of any kind. This point should be stimulated for about 4 minutes until warmth and energy is felt under the finger. This is not always easy to accomplish, especially in obese people, but try your best. You will be amazed what super results will ensue.
4. There are six special acupoints and two hand reflex points for home treatment that can be used to augment the work of Con 6. Sp 9, Sp 6, Ki 6 and Ki 2 are specific points in the treatment of ankle oedema. Each of these points should be stimulated for about 2 minutes on each leg. Be careful when treating patients with congestive heart failure or indeed with any chronic cardiac imbalance – do not stimulate the points with too much enthusiasm. Also, with any oedema, there is bound to be pitting under the fingers that could be very sore to the patient. The other two acupoints are aimed specifically at improving the pericardium energy, which is vital in chronic water retention. They are Bl 14, which is situated between T4 and T5 on the inner bladder line, and P 7 which is located in the middle of the anterior aspect of the wrist crease. An easy energy balance is obtained between P 7 and

Figure 5.10 Points used in oedema.

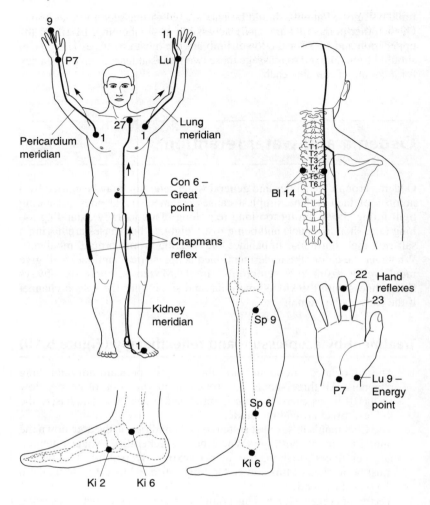

Con 6, but it may be more difficult to obtain a balance between Con 6 and the four lower limb points. Finally, instruct the patient to massage hand reflexes 22 and 23 plus P 7.

5. The energy point is Lu 9 – located just lateral to P 7 on the wrist. This should be stimulated for 2 minutes.

6. Finally, balance the general energy via the Sheng cycle.

Treatment is enhanced if performed with the patient lying with their feet elevated a few inches. This will aid lymphatic and blood circulation.

Hypertension

Definition: Elevation of systolic and/or diastolic blood pressure, either primary (essential hypertension) or secondary to other conditions.

Heredity undoubtedly predisposes individuals to hypertension but the exact mechanism is unclear. Environmental factors (dietary, obesity and stress) seem to act only in genetically susceptible individuals. There is no doubt that stress is a major cause of hypertension. If this is combined with a hectic lifestyle with little relaxation, eating too much salt and processed food and being overweight, the seeds are sown for high blood pressure to present itself. With some people, it can occur very quickly and with others it takes a long time in order for the blood pressure to be so high that action must be taken. Under conditions of rest, a blood pressure reading above 140/90 is considered to indicate hypertension. The chief symptoms are headache, feeling of fullness in the head, dizziness, tinnitus and insomnia. Complications of prolonged untreated hypertension could be stroke, cardiac arrest and asthma. Hypertension is not a condition in its own right; it is merely the body's symptomatic expression of imbalance.

The aims of natural treatment of this syndrome are to provide relaxation (of the body and mind) and to balance, as much as possible, the autonomic nervous system. In TCM terms, the kidney channel has to be stimulated due to kidney Yin. In acupuncture the liver channel is also stimulated but this does not seem to work so well with acupressure. The patient must be prepared to change their lifestyle at the same time that treatment is taking place. It is hopeless to think that acupressure alone can bring down blood pressure if the client is not prepared to change their lifestyle.

Treatment by acupressure and reflextherapy (Figure 5.11)

1. The associated meridian for this syndrome is the small intestine channel. It is a golden rule in acupressure and acupuncture that the heart meridian is never sedated (except in exceptional circumstances). To overcome this, the Yang meridian within the Fire element is used. Stimulating the small intestine has the same effect as sedating the heart. The channel is stroked about 10 times bilaterally in the direction of energy flow.
2. The Chapman's reflexes for the small intestine are situated along the costal margin under the ribs, down the medial aspect of the legs and either side of the mid-thoracic spine. Care should be taken in massaging the costal margin. It can be very tender in cases of hypertension where there are anxiety overtones due to the tension in the solar plexus. It is also extremely tender on the medial side of the legs. Warn the patient!
3. The great point in hypertension is Ki 2. This point is located anterior and inferior to the medial malleolus, in a depression at the anterior and inferior border of the navicular bone. It is one of the more dynamic points on the kidney meridian and is used in strengthening the Yin and dispersing the Yang. The point should be stimulated for up to 4 minutes until heat is produced under the point.
4. There are 11 possible special acupoints and reflex areas that can be used to augment the action of Ki 2. The three points on the medial side of the foot are all concerned with improving the energy in the lower part of the body in order to release the excess at the top. This is useful when the symptoms are headaches, dizziness and tinnitus etc. These points should be stimulated for a couple of minutes each before they are balanced in turn with Ki 2. LI 4 is used extensively in all cases of 'fullness' around the head. The three points on the anterior aspect of

Figure 5.11 Points used in hypertension.

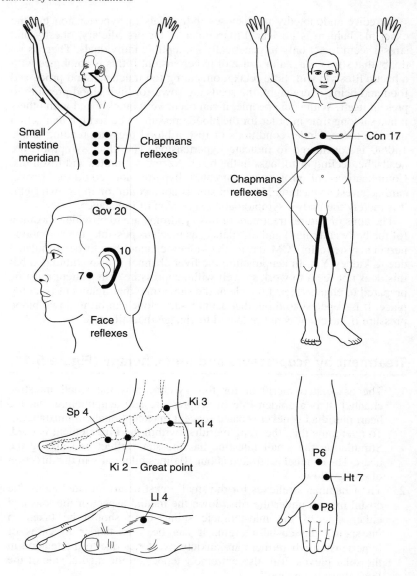

the wrist and hand, P 6, P 8 and Ht 7 are used in different ways to each other. P 6 may be treated if there is general lack of energy, nausea or sickness. Ht 7 is used when there is anxiety and insomnia. P 8 is used in cases of headaches and fullness in the head. It is also a super point for the patient to use at home. It is said to be the hand chakra and has a very similar action to Ki 1 on the sole of the foot in that it reduces headaches, tension and fullness. This point may be balanced with Gov 20 (the crown chakra on top of the head) in order to augment its action. Gov 20 may also be treated in its own right by stretching the scalp apart with the point between the two hands. This is an excellent way of reducing fullness and pressure in the head. Try energy balancing Gov 20 with Ki 2 as a great way to relax the body and mind. For practical purposes, the patient should be sat up with the knees bent up, unless you have very long arms. There is a case here for two-therapist treatment. One therapist holds Gov 20 with the middle finger of the right hand and the other holds Ki 2 with the middle finger of the left hand. Some remarkable results may be had with this method. Con 17, located in the centre of the sternum, I use only when there is tension and anxiety. This point will be discussed fully in the next chapter. Finally, there are two face reflex points, 7 and 10. Area 10 is located around the ear. It should be massaged very lightly. The face points can also be shown to the patient for home treatment. For this, they should be instructed to lie on a comfortable surface with the head lightly supported. They should massage gently around both ears, proceed to gently stimulating point 7, proceeding to Gov 20 and Ht 7. They will then need to sit up in order to massage around the medial aspect of the heel.

5. There is not a suitable energy point for this syndrome. Stimulating Li 3 (in the web between the great and second toes) will help, but the best thing to do is to continue to stimulate the lower kidney points. This can be done in therapy rooms or by the patient at home. He/she can be taught to massage around the whole of the medial aspect of the ankle and heel. It sounds 'hit and miss' but there are so many useful acupoints and reflex points around that area that positive results are bound to ensue.
6. Finally balance the general energy via the Sheng cycle.

Generalized arthritic conditions

The treatment of osteoarthritis was discussed in the last book, but little mention was made of rheumatoid arthritis and, indeed, the treatment of the generalized arthritic syndromes that are so often met in the treatment room. Patients suffering from some form of arthritis probably make up the most common syndrome that therapists are called upon to treat. There are many types of arthritis. The most common two are rheumatoid and osteoarthritis, but others include psoriatic arthritis, infectious arthritis, polychondritis, gout, Reiter's syndrome, Still's disease and ankylosing spondylitis.

Definitions of the most common five:
Rheumatoid arthritis is a chronic syndrome characterized by non-specific, usually symmetric inflammation of the peripheral joints, potentially resulting in progressive destruction of articular and periarticular structures.

Ankylosing spondylitis is a heterogeneous and systemic rheumatic disorder characterized primarily by inflammation of the axial skeleton and large peripheral joints.

Polychondritis is an episodic inflammatory and destructive disorder involving cartilaginous and other connective tissues including ear, joints, nose, larynx, heart valves and blood vessels.

Osteoarthritis is primarily a disorder of hyaline cartilage and subchondral bone, though all tissues in and around involved joints are hypertrophic.

Gout is a recurrent acute arthritis of peripheral joints, which results from deposition, in and about the joints and tendons, of crystals of uric acid. The arthritis may become chronic and deforming.

Some types of arthritis seem to affect individual joints whereas others are systemic diseases that affect the whole of the body's connective tissue. Many theories have been postulated regarding the cause of the different types of arthritis. Probably the most significant factor is, once again, the hereditary factor. Scientific research has now shown that even 'wear and tear' arthritis has a significant hereditary factor. Other causes include faulty eating, lifestyle, gait and posture, virus and bacterial infection, stress and consequences of accidents and injuries. It is also possible that some forms of arthritis may be caused by poison and toxin accumulation from water, food, allergens, inoculations, power cables and other forms of perverse energy and from psychosomatic imbalance. Please remember that the naturopathic way of looking at dis-ease is that it occurs due to the body's response to an internal or external factor. What acupressure and reflextherapy can do is to improve the body's energy levels sufficiently as to fight the offending aetiology. Naturally, if the person insists on eating red meat, denatured flour and sugar, additives and preservatives or engaging in a form of lifestyle that is injurious to clinical progress, there is little that can be achieved by body therapeutics of any kind. It is totally up to the patient, in these and any other conditions, to want to be well. Patients have to meet the therapist half way – they cannot expect a magic wand to be waved to cure their entire ills whilst they are still in a destructive mode of action and thought.

Treatment by acupressure and reflextherapy (Figure 5.12)

1. The associated meridian is the kidney channel. This is because the kidney is responsible for our ancestral energy and, as most arthritis is based on hereditary factors, this channel has to be energy boosted. Also by improving the kidney energy, the adrenal glands are stimulated, thus helping with the liberation of cortisone, which aids pain relief and mobility. The channel needs to be stroked bilaterally about 10 times in the flow of energy from the foot towards the upper chest.
2. The Chapman's reflex areas for the kidney are located on the chest and abdomen front and the large triangular area above the sacrum. In such a systemic condition as arthritis, it is far better to massage all the reflexes. It only takes a couple of minutes and is so much better.
3. There are no great and energy points as such; instead there is a routine or 'formula' of treatment for both the acute/sub-acute and chronic forms of arthritis. There are also a few special points. The key in arthritis, as mentioned before, is to liberate the patient's own cortisone. This is quite a complex thing to do, but once the technique is mastered it will be your saviour over and over again. The hormone cortisone comes from the adrenal cortex, which in turn is controlled by the gonadotrophic centre of the anterior pituitary gland, which produces adrenocorticotrophic hormone (ACTH). The formula is to stimulate the point Bl 1, followed by stimulating the key points of the eight extra meridians, followed by stimulating the base chakra. (I shall not dwell on describing the various chakras and their particular significance in hormonal release because a book on the subject will be forthcoming.)

Figure 5.12 Points used in generalized arthritis.

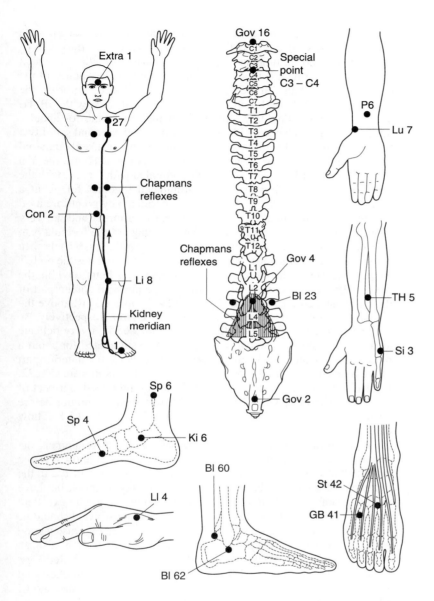

When practising acupuncture, the point Bl 1 may be used to stimulate the anterior pituitary. Bl 1 is positioned about a centimetre deep to the inner canthus of the eye. It isn't a favourite point of many acupuncturists due to its location. It is, obviously, impossible to massage the point. Several years ago, I invented an acupressure alternative based upon stimulating the Ajna chakra points together with the key points of the Ajna chakra, Sp 6 and Gov 4. The Ajna chakra points are Extra 1 (Yintang), located between the eyes; and Gov 16, located in the midline between the occiput and atlas. These two points are stimulated and balanced with each other. This should take a couple of minutes to achieve. Then stimulate Gov 4, located between L2 and L3, for a minute and balance it with Extra 1. Finally, stimulate Sp 6, located 3 cun above the medial malleolus, for a minute and balance it with Extra 1. This triad of points is the equivalent of piercing Bl 1 and starting the process of pituitary stimulation. The next stage of the treatment is to stimulate and balance the key points of the eight extra meridians. In the case of acute and sub-acute arthritis, the points are Si 3 balanced with Bl 62 and TH 5 balanced with GB 41. The two couples should be stimulated at the same time for about a minute and then balanced with each other before the second set of two points are treated. In all cases of chronic osteoarthritis, rheumatoid arthritis and ankylosing spondylitis, the key points used are the Yin ones of Ki 6 coupled with Lu 7 and Sp 4 coupled with P 6. As with the Yang ones, these points should be stimulated together for about a minute before balancing. The eight extra meridian key points are used extensively in acupuncture in the treatment of arthritis and are very adaptable to use with acupressure. The next stage of the formula is to stimulate and balance the points associated with the base chakra. In some ways, this is the most important stage, as it stimulates the body's deepest energies, namely the ancestral energy that is housed within the base chakra. The two points that comprise the physical counterpart of the base chakra are Con 2 and Gov 2. They are located just above the symphysis pubis and between the coccyx and sacrum, respectively. Be very careful how they are treated; they are located in a very delicate area of the anatomy. The two points should be stimulated for about a minute and balanced. It is only necessary to balance the anterior part of the base chakra with the two key points. The key points are Con 22, located in the sternal notch, and Li 8, located on the medial aspect of the knee. Stimulate Con 2 and Con 22 for about a minute before balancing them. Stimulating and balancing Con 2 with Li 8 follow this.

4.   There are some special points that may also be used to augment the above procedure. There is a point located between C3 and C4 in the midline that was taught to me over 25 years ago as being of use in the treatment of arthritis. I have never found it in any textbook but have used it steadfastly in both acupuncture and acupressure with excellent results. It seems to affect the neck and shoulders mostly and should be stimulated for at least 2 minutes to have any effect. Bl 23 is also a good point to use when kidney energy is to be stimulated. It is also an excellent point to create energy and dispel tiredness and lethargy. Finally, there are the classical pain relief points of LI 4 – chest and shoulders, St 42 – ankle, Bl 60 – foot and ankle, Bl 40 – knee and LI 15 – shoulder. Information on these points is given in the previous book.

5.   It is always favourable to complete the treatment with a general energy balance via the Sheng cycle.

The treatment outlined for generalized arthritis may seem to be long-winded and tedious. In actual fact, in practice, it is not. It does, though, afford the bodyworker an excellent opportunity to treat some of the most painful and crippling of conditions that are seen on a regular basis, without the need to use electrotherapy or to be reliant on suppressant drugs. A full list breakdown of how to use acupressure to liberate other hormones (adrenaline, thyroxine and oestrogen) as well as a full explanation of the liberation of cortisone will be given in the next publication.

Hemiplegia (hemiparesis)

Definition: A cerebrovascular accident (CVA) of an important section of the brain's arterial system that gives rise to pain, stiffness and loss of movement of the opposite side of the body. The blood vessel that regularly bursts is the lenticulo-striate branch of the middle cerebral artery. Although it is more common in the over 50s, it can occur in children. The cause is unknown, but the hereditary factor seems to be strong. In TCM terms, there is an invasion of Fong (Wind) that penetrates the body and affects mostly the liver, stomach and gall bladder meridians. The aim of any treatment is therefore aimed at moving Chi and blood and eliminating Wind. In Western terms, this means reducing muscle spasm and restoring co-ordination of the affected limb. In recent times, the use of acupuncture has been seen in physiotherapy departments to supplement the orthodox methods of exercise and movement therapy. I have been using acupressure and reflextherapy in stroke victims for several years and present the following as being a purely subjective viewpoint. Acupressure in isolation, though, will not treat the whole person. Physical rehabilitation consisting of kinesiology and movement therapy combined with the specialized techniques of Bobath, Rood and proprioceptive neuromuscular facilitation (PNF) all have their place.

Treatment by acupressure and reflextherapy (Figure 5.13)

1. The associated meridians are the liver, gall bladder and stomach channels. These need to be stroked in the direction of energy flow about 10 times each. Special emphasis should be given to the areas of the meridians that lie on the affected limb.
2. The Chapman's reflex areas lie underneath the pectoralis major muscles and either side of the lower end of the sternum. These should be massaged with stimulation, although, as has been stated on many occasions, it would be far better to massage them all. This could, though, present logistical problems due to the possible inability of the patient to move freely in order to receive treatment.
3. The great point is GB 34. This point is located in the depression anterior and inferior to the head of fibula. It is said to be *the* great point in musculo-tendinous conditions and specifically acts on reducing muscle spasm. Because of the chronicity of this condition, the point should be massage bilaterally (affected and non-affected legs) for up to 5 minutes. This will stir the gall bladder and liver Chi into action in preparation for the remainder of the treatment session.
4. There are six sets of special points, depending on where the stroke has affected the patient. They are located on the head, hand, foot, front of body, arm and leg. *Treatment of an affected arm* – Con 22 is stimulated for up to 2 minutes in order to bring Chi to the front of the chest, throat and back of the neck. This should be followed, in turn, by stimulating LI 15, LI 11 and LI 4 each for about 2 minutes. With each subsequent stimulation, the affected arm should feel slightly warmer and pliant. It would be of enormous help to be able to balance each of the arm points with GB 34; this really enhances the treatment. The patient will often

Figure 5.13 Points used in hemiplegia.

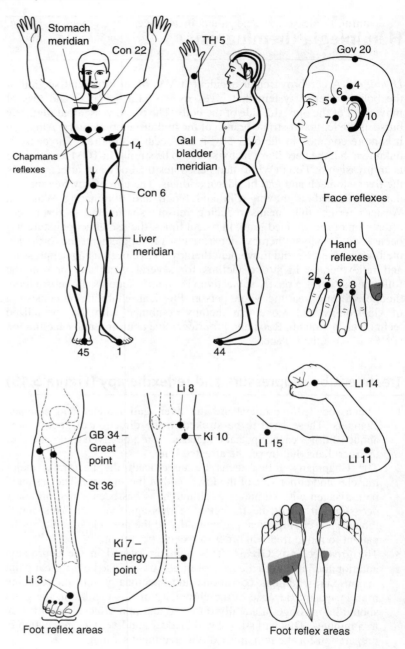

remark that they feel 'electricity' being stirred up inside them. They often feel tingling and glowing where before the limb had appeared dead. This is, in no way, to indicate that acupressure can cure hemiplegia – of course it can't. It is, though, capable of enabling the affected limb to feel more bearable and less painful for the patient. This can be followed by treatment of hand reflexes 2, 4, 6 and 8 and the area around the thumb. The reflexes are often called ah-shi points and are located on the 'v' of the finger webs. They can be quite painful, so please warn the patient in advance. They can also be taught to massage these points themselves. The thumb reflex area is associated with the head and can be quite useful if the patient massages it regularly. *Treatment of an affected leg* – Con 6 should be stimulated for up to 3 minutes sufficient as to bring Chi to the area. This should be followed, in turn, by stimulating the following points – St 36, Li 8/Ki 10, Li 3. Each should be stimulated for 2 minutes and be balanced with GB 34 afterwards. Li 8 and Ki 10 are located so close to each other on the medial aspect of the knee that they are often considered as being one point (in acupressure terms). Following the stimulation and balancing of Li 3 with GB 34, the ah-shi points on the feet may be stimulated. They lie in the 'v' of the webs on the toes. Whilst the foot ah-shi points are being treated, it would be advantageous to treat the foot reflex points associated with the liver, gall bladder and head. The foot pattern is also used in the treatment of affected arms as well. *Treatment using head points* – The five reflex points and one acupoint on the head are used after the treatment of either or both of the affected limbs. Personal experience has shown that these points represent some of the most effective in the whole of bodywork. Point 7 and area 10 are used for high blood pressure (which may have triggered off the CVA in the first place). These two points need to be gently massaged for anything up to 3 minutes. Treating points 5, 6 and 4, in that order, should follow. They are used for 'brain fog', relaxation of muscles and relaxation of the mind, respectively. These points should not be stimulated. If they are, it is likely that symptoms will be made worse. The ideal way to treat these points is to stand or sit behind the patient and gently place the middle fingers of both hands on each point in turn for about two to 3 minutes. Sedating Gov 20 using the scalp stretching method previously described may follow this. This important head treatment often enables the patient to think more clearly and to feel more self-confident, which is a great boon to them. These points may also be used in the symptomatic treatment of other neurological conditions. Try it – it works!

5. The energy point is Ki 7. It is important to stimulate this point for up to 2 minutes following the main part of the session in order not to 'lose' the body Chi that has been gained. Warn the patient that they may feel sleepy following the treatment session.
6. Finally, balance the general body energy via the Sheng cycle.

The treatment of hemiplegia with acupressure and reflextherapy should give the therapist a template as to the treatment of other neurological conditions. The head points remain the same, the peripheral points are chosen as to the symptoms presented. Please remember that you are not curing these conditions. You are, though, making a huge difference to many of the patient's symptoms as well as their outlook and confidence.

Chronic fatigue syndrome

Definition: A weakening of the immune system giving rise to lethargy, muscular pain and headaches. Other symptoms may include dizziness, depression, nausea, poor appetite, chest pains and backaches. The syndrome is also known as post-viral syndrome, myalgic encephalo-myelitis (ME), Epstein–Barr syndrome or yuppie flu. It came to prominence in the 1980s, when it was generally discarded by physicians as being a psychosomatic disorder. It was often called 'lazy teenager syndrome' or yuppie flu, because symptoms usually followed contracting some kind of virus. It was only in the middle 1990s that it was recognized as a definite condition. The diagnosis is very difficult because it is multi-factorial in its aetiology and presenting symptoms. The possible causes are viral infection, eating faulty food for many years, sequelae of a shock to the system (as in a car accident or emotional trauma) or as a result of more than one of these and other factors. There is a weakening of the immune system that enables the virus to thrive, which in turn weakens the immune system more, thus producing a vicious circle. My own amateur research, compiled after having treated scores of patients who had been labelled with this condition came to the following conclusions: 80% had a violent reaction, as babies, to one or more inoculation or vaccination; 85% had suffered from glandular fever as adolescents; 97% had indeed suffered from a 'flu' like virus weeks or months before the symptoms of chronic fatigue syndrome (CFS) started. Lastly but not least, there was a significant percentage – 71% – that had been born by Caesarean section. This data would indicate to me that the patient had been subject to some kind of trauma, and there is nothing so traumatic as birth trauma. I hope to carry out more research on the subject, as time allows.

In her book, *Acupuncture in Clinical Practice*, Nadia Ellis describes the symptoms in TCM terms as follows:

- Excess conditions:
  - Fatigue, aching muscles, lack of concentration and muzziness. Tongue – sticky yellow coating, pulse – slippery, as being due to *damp-heat in the muscles*.
  - Muscle fatigue without pain, thirst, insomnia, breathlessness and cough with scanty yellow sputum and weight loss. Tongue – red with a yellow coating, pulse – rapid and wiry, as being due to *heat in the interior*.

- Deficient conditions:
  - Fatigue worse at the start of the day, lack of vital energy, shortness of breath, sweating during the day, poor appetite and loose stools. Tongue – pale, pulse – empty as being due to *Chi deficiency*.

In the more chronic and long-lasting cases, there appears to be Yin deficiency in the lung, stomach and kidney, which can give rise to various symptoms – exhaustion, cough, night sweats, dry mouth, tinnitus, insomnia and even deafness.

The reader can easily see that whether the condition is described in traditional or modern terms, the symptoms presented vary enormously. This can often make it difficult to diagnose and treat with any form of medicine, let alone with bodywork.

Treatment by acupressure and reflextherapy (Figure 5.14)

Treatment is naturally determined by the symptoms presented, but the overall aim is to use the body's energy system to improve the quality and quantity of Chi in the immune system, liver, spleen and kidney (the three

Figure 5.14 Points used in chronic fatigue syndrome.

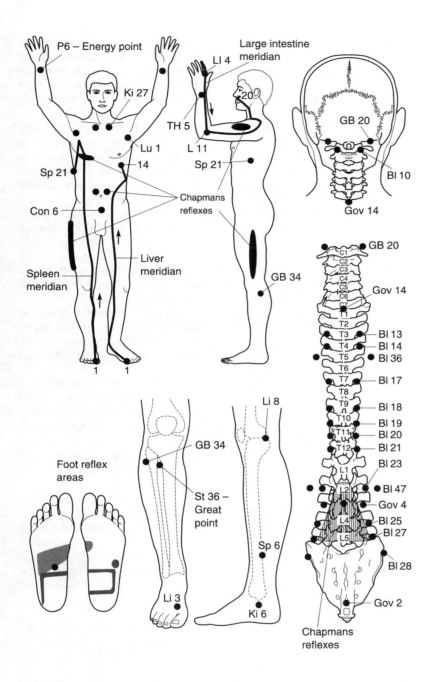

Leg–Yin meridians and the ones most affected in CFS). The large intestine channel is also used due to its action in excretion of toxins etc.

1. The associated meridians are the spleen, liver and large intestine. They should each be stroked bilaterally in the direction of energy flow about 10 times each. Emphasis should be made around the command points areas between the toes and knee and the fingers and elbow.
2. The Chapman's reflexes are very important in the treatment of this condition. The muscles are invariably sluggish and stiff and need their

lymph and blood circulation stimulated. The areas are to be found under the right pectoralis muscle, either side of the umbilicus, down the lateral aspect of the leg, above the sacrum and underneath the deltoid insertion on the arm. This, though, is definitely one condition when massaging all the Chapman's reflexes will really benefit the patient.

3. The great point is St 36. This is because, of all the points in the body, it is the one that improves the general energy pattern most of all – in other words it creates Chi where before there was a deficiency. This point should be stimulated for about 5 minutes. This is no mean feat – it is a long time. If the patient starts to feel nauseous, either ease back on the amount of stimulation or cease altogether.

4. There are scores of special points and should be used dependent on the presenting symptoms. It is not necessary to use all the points suggested below.

    In all cases
    - The foot reflexes associated with the liver, gall bladder, spleen and large intestine should be massaged either in isolation or as part of a general foot reflexology treatment pattern.
    - Sp 6 – located 3 cun superior to the medial malleolus should be stimulated for about 2 minutes before it is balanced with St 36. Sp 6 is located at the point in the leg where the three channels of liver, kidney and spleen cross. It is possible, therefore, to stimulate all three channels using this one point.
    - The back transporting points should each be stimulated, although they could have been treated earlier whilst doing a generalized Chapman's reflex pattern. They all lie in the inner bladder line, with the exception of Bl 36 and Bl 47, which are located in the outer bladder line. Massaging the back transporting points is a wonderful way of improving the general energy quantity in the organs themselves. See Figure 3.5 for the related organs.

    To treat muscle pain and stiffness
    - Li 3 is used to treat muscle cramps and stiffness. It is also an excellent point for general stress and clearing the mind.
    - GB 34 is used to promote the smooth flow of liver and gall bladder Chi. It is an important point in relaxing tendons and muscles, especially where there is a damp-heat situation.
    - GB 20 and Bl 10 are used to relax the tension in the cervical muscles and the back of the head. They are also used in the treatment of headaches.

    To stimulate the immune system
    - Sp 21 is located in the sixth intercostal space in the mid-axillary line. It is said to be the general connecting point of the Yang meridians. It is useful in moving 'stuck' Chi in the muscles and spleen and helps with the general lymphatic and blood circulation. Please note that this point is very sensitive in the majority of people, and is extra painful when it needs treatment. The patient must be warned.
    - Con 6 and Gov 4 are stimulated together. They form the anterior and posterior aspects of the sacral chakra, which is concerned with the immune system as well as dealing with water and lymph balance. Ideally, the patient should be in side lying so as to get to both points. They should be stimulated for about 2 minutes; then Con 6 should be balanced with St 36.

- Bl 23 and Bl 47 were mentioned in the section in treating all cases. They have specific influence in the improvement of the immune system in that they improve the general kidney and adrenal energy and help in the liberation of adrenaline and cortisone.
- Li 8 is located at the medial end of the knee joint. It has great influence in removing damp conditions and also to nourish and tonify the blood. It is also the key point to the base chakra and has an influence in helping with depression and lifting the spirits.

To aid excretion of toxins
- The main points to use are LI 4 and LI 11. These should both be stimulated for 2 minutes before balancing with St 36.

Other points
- Ki 6, located inferior to the medial malleolus, is a major point of influence in this condition. It is widely used in Yin deficiency. It helps clear the eyes and head. It also calms the mind and helps clear any throat congestion that may occur.
- TH 5, located 2 cun superior to the posterior wrist crease, is used in the treatment of fullness in the head (combined with LI 4 and GB 20) and for heat and sweating. It is a major point for releasing wind-heat due to infection.
- Ki 27, located just inferior to the medial aspect of the clavicle, and Lu 1, located 2 cun lateral to the nipple line in the second intercostal space, are both used when there is chest congestion, tightness and muscular tension of the respiratory muscles.

5. The energy point is P 6. As well as being a good tonification for the spleen meridian and the immune system, it has a powerful calming action on the mind if there is any anxiety present. It should be stimulated for a minute before being balanced with St 36. This represents a very powerful balance in this condition.
6. Finally, the general body energy should be balanced via the Sheng cycle.

Owing to the complexity of CFS, it is not always possible to get as much satisfaction in its treatment as with some conditions. Some patients react far better than others. What acupressure and reflextherapy achieve that no other form of therapy comes close to doing is the combination of energy, immune system, muscle weakness, excretion and lymphatic flow improvement. The points described may be used for a myriad of similar syndromes.

Migraine and chronic headaches

Definition: A paroxysmal disorder characterized by recurrent attacks of headache, with or without associated visual and digestive disturbances. The symptoms are various depending on the cause. Headaches can occur in all areas of the head, be of different types of pain and have secondary influences on the vision, bladder and stomach. Some people accept headaches as a normal by-product of their lifestyles; others rush for the aspirin the minute that they have a twinge of pain, others still do not know what it is like to suffer from them. The aetiology is sometimes complicated and they often occur due to more than one factor. Each case has to be treated on its own merit as an individual and unique case. This is one aspect of natural therapy where two patients can describe exactly the same symptoms and yet have totally different causes and subsequent treatment. Always examine thoroughly and never assume the findings in advance – there is often a surprise to be had. The following observations represents my personal findings over many years of practice of the many causes of migraine and chronic headaches.

The most common cause of a chronic headache (and sometimes migraine) is muscular tension in the sub-occipital muscles. This can occur due to everyday stress and tension, bad posture or by increased inter-cranial pressure due to high blood pressure. This type of headache usually affects the frontal part of the head over the eyes. It is easy to treat by localized acupressure and distal foot and hand reflextherapy.

The next most common cause of headaches and *the* most common cause of migraine occur as a result of a cervical lesion. It has never ceased to amaze me over the years of treating this condition of the high percentage of patients who present with a neck lesion. Quite often these people have been fobbed off with analgesics for several years, even had scans and X-rays, and yet not been correctly diagnosed. The secret, as always, of discerning whether or not there is a cervical lesion is to *ask*. Cervical lesions don't just happen; they usually follow a whiplash or some other kind of trauma. They can occur as a child, with banging the head or falling onto the heels causing a ricochet vibration towards the head and subsequent mis-alignment or displacement of a vertebra at an age when the joints and tendons are extremely vulnerable. It is only when the person reaches the age of 18 or so those symptoms often start. It is hopeless in the extreme to give acupressure or any other form of natural medicine for a headache if the correct treatment lies in mechanical adjustment by a recognized practitioner. Therefore if you feel that there is an underlying vertebral anomaly, and you are an osteopath, chiropractor or manipulative physiotherapist, then adjust it! If you do not possess manipulative skills, refer the patient to someone who has. Details of how to adjust cervical vertebrae using very gentle methods that utilize the energy system are to be found in the book on the treatment of musculo-skeletal conditions. Diplopia, flashing lights and zigzags often accompany this type of headache and migraine, especially if there is atlas and cranial base involvement.

Faulty eating is a common cause of headaches and migraine. Eating too much fatty food may upset the gall bladder, which in turn may give rise to hemi-cranial headaches. There is often nausea and vomiting with this type and the pain is very sharp and piercing. Treatment concentrates on taking tension out of the gall bladder and liver. Eating too much saturated fat, denatured sugar and flour and preservatives may clog the bowel and give rise to general pain headaches of the 'sick' kind. Treatment consists of using local points and those along the large intestine meridian. Sometimes faulty eating affects the stomach as well as the large bowel. This produces a more severe headache, usually centred over the eyes and around the St 8 point just under the hair-line. The treatment uses mostly points on the stomach meridian. A common reason for headache and migraine is for the person to consume a particular food to saturation level over several years, thus creating an integral toxic situation. The symptomatic expression of headache will ensue each time that the 'trigger' food is eaten. The most common trigger foods are chocolate, cheese, oranges, wine and tomatoes. In each and every case of migraine and headache being caused by eating too much or by eating the wrong foods, it goes without saying that the patient *must* abstain from those foods.

A common cause of headache is by being subjected to a cold wind. This often affects the frontal part of the head. Treatment consists of using local head points and by strengthening the liver meridian, which makes the person less susceptible to be afflicted, and easily cures it.

An ever-increasing cause of headache is caused by reaction to perverse energy. This can arise from handling mobile phones, sitting in front of a monitor, using a photocopier or by using a myriad of different electronic gadgets. This type of headache is more difficult to treat. It consists of using local head points plus hand and foot reflex points.

A more chronic form of headache may arise due to liver energy imbalance over a period of years. The aetiology is uncertain although reactions to viruses, possibly several years previously is very common. This is the 'liver Yang rising' pain (in TCM terms) that can give classical migraine symptoms of chronic sharp pain which is worse for movement, noise and smells. The patient must lie down, be quiet and lie onto the painful side. They also feel dizzy and sick. Treatment consists of balancing liver and stomach energy.

Stress and tension can produce constant niggling headaches. Treatment is by acupressure, gentle massage around the neck and shoulders, a good hot bath and TLC. Maintaining personal fitness of the body *and* mind is also a paramount factor in the treatment rationale.

Patients often present with headaches that arise as secondary symptoms to other conditions. Treatment will vary with the cause.

Treatment by acupressure and reflextherapy (Figure 5.15)

1. The associated meridians are the liver and gall bladder. These should be stroked in the direction of energy flow about 10 times each. When the pain is acute, they should be stroked against the flow of energy the same number of times.
2. The related Chapman's reflexes are situated under the right pectoralis major muscle, either side of the lower sternum and under the left clavicle.
3. There are two great points – LI 4 and Li 3. The reader will have noticed that these two points often work in tandem. As has been mentioned in a previous chapter, they are, in fact, the same point, being positioned in exactly the same place on the hand and foot. They are excellent points to stimulate in the first instance of treating headaches and migraine because they provide a relaxing, calming and analgesic effect within a couple of minutes. The ideal way to use the points is to stimulate each for 2 minutes and then create a balance between the two. Please note that LI 4 should not be stimulated in pregnancy or in the first 2 days of menstruation. If this is the case, Li 3 may be used in isolation.
4. There are several special points that can be used to augment the action of LI 4 and Li 3. They may be broken down into the following areas: local head reflex and acupoints, hand reflex points, foot reflex and acupoints and there are four miscellaneous points. All treatment should take place with the patient in lying.

Figure 5.15 Points used in migraine.

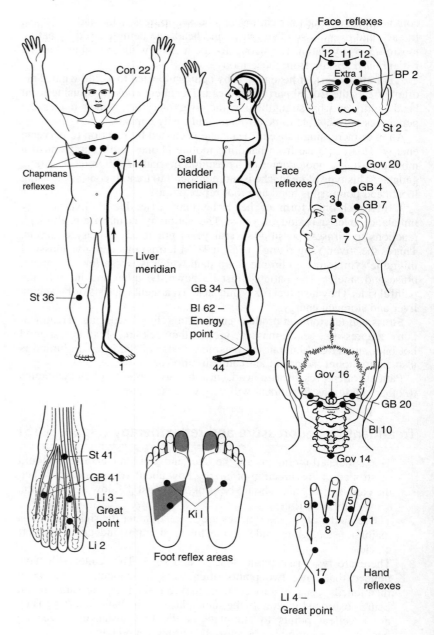

- The head acupoints and reflex points may be treated in isolation or in combination with a suitable distal point. Extra 1 and Gov 16 are used in tandem to help clear the head of 'fog' and to calm the mind. Reflex points 11 and 12 are used in frontal headaches and when there is blurred vision. Take care to stimulate the points sufficiently as to create some energy under the fingers, after this they should be sedated and balanced with LI 4. Point 11 is particularly effective when there is a great frontal pressure build up. Reflex point 7 is also used in pressure headaches; particularly

those caused by high blood pressure. Reflex point 5 is used as a
great calming point and for clearing 'brain fog'. It is positioned on
the Pterion where the greater wing of the sphenoid bone can be
felt. It is said to have a direct access to the hypothalamus and can,
of course, be used in many other conditions other than headache –
see Chapter 6. Reflex point 3 lies about 1 cun superior to point 5
and is used in cases of double vision and pressure headaches.
Reflex point 1 lies on the Bregma, on the division between the
parietals and the frontal bone. It is an excellent point for pressure
headaches, especially those when the top of the head seems to be
bursting. The point may be sedated, stretched using both hands or
balanced with LI 4. There are seven meridian acupoints that are
useful. GB 4 and GB 7 are useful in the treatment of hemi-cranial
headaches and sick headaches. These two points should never be
stimulated. The best way to use them is to sedate them and balance
them with either LI 4 or a distal point on the gall bladder meridian
– either GB 34 by the knee or GB 41 on the foot. Gov 20 is used
as a general point to relax the mind and to ease tension. It is the
physical counterpart of the crown chakra – known as the thousand
petalled lotus or the point of a thousand meetings. It is an excellent
calming point. One word of warning about this point: make sure
your patient is lying down when this point is being treated. If it is
over-treated it can cause the patient to feel 'spaced out' or even
faint. It should be handled very carefully and if your patient tells
you they are feeling slightly faint, gently take the hand away. Bl 2
is useful for the treatment of eye strain, sinusitis and frontal
headaches. This point also should not be stimulated but balanced
either with LI 4 or Bl 62 on the outside of the ankle (long arms
needed here). St 2 is used in eyestrain and in headaches caused by
stomach imbalance. It is also used in the localized treatment of
sinusitis. It should be balanced either with LI 4 or with St 36. This
is an excellent point in the treatment of hyperactivity – see Chapter
6. The two points on the posterior aspect of the head – GB 20 and
Bl 10 – have been discussed before as being superb points in the
treatment of head and neck tension. They are always tender when
a headache is around and represent very good self-treatment points
that are easily accessible. When the therapist is doing the
treatment, these points are best used by energy balancing them
with either LI 4 or TH 5.

- There are six hand reflex points that can be used by the patient in
  self-treatment (plus LI 4). Reflex point 1 is used for occipital
  (posterior) headaches, reflex point 5 is used for pressure headaches
  in the cranium, reflex points 7 and 9 are used for frontal headaches,
  reflex point 8 is used for neck pains and reflex point 17 is used in
  sinusitis. This may seem rather confusing at first but, as in all
  things, practice makes perfect. Each point should be used as *bona
  fide* distal points and should be used in energy balancing.
- The foot reflex areas marked on Figure 5.15 are associated with the
  liver, gall bladder and head. These areas should be supplemented
  with any other areas that the therapist feels will be effective, e.g.
  stomach, kidney, spleen, cervical etc. The three acupoints on the
  foot besides Li 3 are Li 2, GB 41 and St 41. Li 2 is a very good
  distal point in 'liverish' headaches due to overeating and
  hangovers. GB 41 and St 41 are both distal points used either in

isolation or in combination with local points. GB 41 is the best distal point in hemi-cranial headaches and St 41 is useful to help with headaches caused by eating or drinking cold food or drink.

- Con 22 and Gov 14 may be used in tandem to help release tension in the lower cervical region and shoulders in order to ease occipital and frontal headaches. This combination is also used in headaches caused by people having constipation or food intolerance. St 36 may be used as a distal point to supplement the use of St 2 on the head. It may also be used in isolation as a distal point in the treatment of 'sick' headaches and nausea. It is also one of the best 'energy giving' points in the body and should be used to help restore energy balance following a prolonged period of headaches. GB 34 may be used as a distal point alongside GB 4 and GB 7 or in isolation as a distal point to help with muscular spasm of the occipital and scalp muscles occurring in headaches.

5. The energy point is Bl 62, located just inferior to the lateral malleolus. This point should be stimulated for about 2 minutes.
6. Finally, balance the general body energy via the Sheng cycle.

Insomnia

Definition: Difficulty in sleeping or a disturbed sleep pattern leading to the perception of insufficient sleep. Insomnia is a common symptom and may be due to several emotional and physical disorders. With advancing age, the total amount of sleep tends to shorten. Initial insomnia (difficulty in falling asleep) is commonly associated with an emotional disturbance such as anxiety, a phobic state, or depression. In early morning awakening, the patient falls asleep normally but awakens several hours before his or her usual time and either cannot fall asleep again or drifts into a restless unsatisfying sleep. An inverted sleep rhythm may develop in elderly people because of inappropriate use of sedatives, often prescribed for insomnia. It is rare, though not impossible, for a patient to present him/herself to the therapist just with insomnia. It often occurs as an 'also ran' and is something that they accept as being 'normal'. Constant insomnia can, though, cause havoc with lifestyle and whether or not our energy levels are maintained. It can also be a well-known side effect of drug medication, which then leads to further prescriptions of sleep-inducing drugs being prescribed. Insomnia may also be purely symptomatic of a deeper problem. Treatment by acupressure helps relax the body and mind in order to regain a normal sleep pattern. In so doing, it very often brings to the fore the original dis-ease pattern which has caused it in the first place.

Treatment by acupressure and reflextherapy (Figure 5.16)

1. The associated meridian is the pericardium channel. This needs to be stroked bilaterally with the flow of energy about 10 times. Extra emphasis should be made on the area between the fingers and elbow.
2. There are no Chapman's reflexes for this condition.

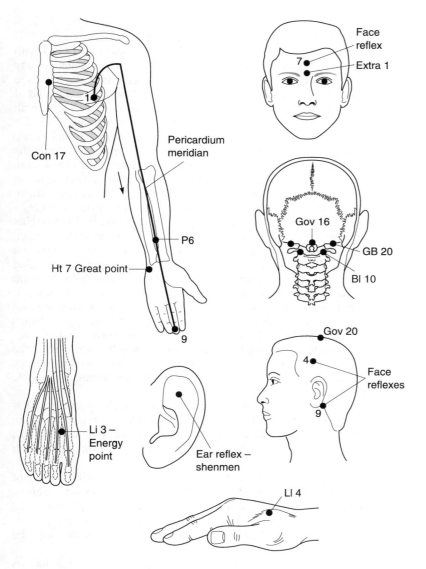

Figure 5.16 Points used in insomnia.

3. The great point in this condition is Ht 7. It is located on the medial aspect of the anterior wrist crease just proximal to the pisiform bone. This point should be stimulated for about 2 minutes, after which a warmth and relaxation should be felt. Continued stimulation should induce relaxation and sleep. This point is easily positioned for patients to use it themselves whilst in bed.

4. There are a number of special points that can be used in order to reinforce the action of Ht 7. They are positioned on the head and neck, chest, arm and ear.
   - **Head and neck points** – There are five acupoints and three face reflex points that can be used in insomnia. They may all be used in self-treatment and each has a slightly different mode of action. Following the stimulation of Ht 7, the most effective head point to

use is head reflex point 7. This point, shown in Figure 3.17, is located one-third the way up between Extra 1 and the hairline. It is a traditional point in insomnia and is said to have a direct link with the psyche. This point should be sedated, not stimulated in any way. If the patient is doing the treatment, make sure that he or she has their arm supported at the elbow so that they can keep hold of the point for the 3 or 4 minutes that is necessary to produce an effective treatment. The same practical advice holds water for sedating the other facial points, it is useless to try and create relaxation that is a precursor to sleep if the arm that is doing the treatment is in spasm. The two other face reflex points are useful, though not so effective as no. 7. Point no. 4 is very good in relaxing the mind from any extraneous thoughts prior to treatment and point 9 is more for relaxation of the upper cervical muscles – which is also important. The acupoints GB 20 and Bl 10 also relax the post-cervical muscles as well as easing tension in the occiput. These two points should be gently massaged prior to holding them for up to 2 minutes. The best duo of points, though, for inducing relaxation and for clearing the mind is Gov 16 coupled with Extra 1. These points have been mentioned before as being the anterior and posterior components of the brow (Ajna) chakra. They are said to have a direct link with the pituitary gland and the hypothalamus region of the brain. Hold these two points for about 2 or 3 minutes to experience amazing relaxation. Gov 20 may be used to relax the whole of the body and to clear the mind. An excellent energy balance may be obtained with Ht 7, though it is almost impossible to do this on oneself.

- **Chest** – Con 17 is located in the centre of the sternum and is always tender when needed to be treated. This point is excellent in the treatment of anxiety and the irritation and frustration of not being able to sleep. Stimulate it first for a minute, then balance it with Ht 7.
- **Arm** – P 6 is one of the best points to treat the possible causes of insomnia. These include headache, anxiety, palpitations, nausea, indigestion and general malaise. The point should be stimulated for about 2 minutes. LI 4 should be used if there is any pain or discomfort in the head, chest, throat or shoulders that may be contributing to the insomnia.
- **Ear** – The ear is an unusual reflex area to use and it has its limitations in acupressure. One of the best-known points and most widely used is point Shenmen. This famous point may be used in cases of anxiety, stress, tension and brain fog. I find it particularly useful when the brain appears to be 'jumbled up' and needs clearing – good for students studying for an exam. If the therapist treats the point, it is best to use a baby bud or the end of a matchstick with some cotton wool attached. In self-treatment, the little finger should be used. The TCM word Shenmen (or spirit gate) is also the term for point Ht 7, so the two points seem to be ideally suited.

5. The energy point in this condition is Li 3. It is an excellent 'finishing' point because it helps relax the body and mind. Do not use this in self-treatment, as it is slightly awkward to reach and stay relaxed at the same time.
6. Finally, balance the body's energy via the Sheng cycle.

Acupressure 'maintenance' therapy

It is rare indeed to meet an adult who has not suffered from some kind of dis-ease in their lives. Very many illnesses that people suffer from can, in the main, be prevented by regularly and routinely doing an acupressure work-out routine. Young and old may carry out the undermentioned procedure with disregard for the individual underlying condition. Acupressure and reflextherapy treat the whole person and not just individual conditions, therefore if the energy system or Chi is balanced and maintained, it should prevent many of the diseases that we all regularly suffer from. The system is my own invention and is based upon balancing the Hara (Con 6) with many of the body's vital organs and functions. It is made simple so that it may be easily undertaken, and it is made practically easy so as not to tie oneself into knots with self-treatment (Figure 5.17).

- Lie down on a comfortable surface with the head slightly raised on a pillow. With the middle finger pad of the right hand stimulate Con 6 (two finger widths below the umbilicus (navel)) for about 1 minute; this should be done gently but firmly.
- Bend up the knees. With the middle finger pad of the left hand, gently stimulate St 36. This point is located one finger-breadth lateral to the tibial tubercle. This should be massaged for about 1 minute. Now energy balance the two points by keeping the fingers still for a further 2 minutes.

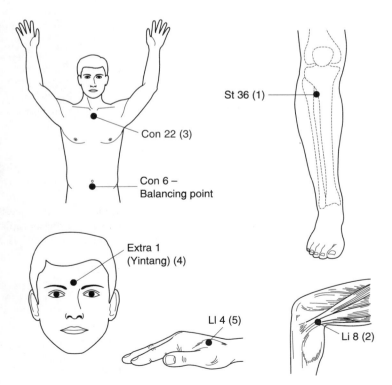

Figure 5.17 Points used in acupressure maintenance therapy.

St 36 (1)

Con 22 (3)

Con 6 – Balancing point

Extra 1 (Yintang) (4)

LI 4 (5)

Li 8 (2)

- With the right middle finger still on Con 6, transfer the left hand over to gently stimulate Li 8 on the right knee. This point is located on the very medial aspect of the knee. Again, massage it for a minute and energy balance it with Con 6.
- Now transfer the left middle finger to Con 22, situated in the sternal notch. Repeat the procedure of gentle stimulation and energy balancing.
- Take the left hand now to Extra 1, positioned between the eyes, and repeat the procedure.
- Finally, gently stimulate LI 4 on the right hand (still holding Con 6 with the middle finger), then balance the two points for a couple of minutes.

This procedure takes about 10–15 minutes and should be carried out during a relaxation period about once a week. The initial reaction to the treatment will be tiredness, relaxation and a feeling of well being. The more the system is used, the more the recipient will find that general aches and pains, stresses and temper will all be improved.

6

Treatment of stress, emotional and mental conditions

Stress-related conditions, emotional imbalance and some mild mental symptoms answer very well to treatment by acupressure and reflextherapy. It represents a real alternative to drug therapy, psychotherapy and hypnotherapy. The wonderful therapeutic and relaxation effects of touch and massage have already been pointed out in an earlier chapter. There is an increasing tolerance towards the acceptance and subsequent treatment of emotional conditions. When I started clinical practice, it was extremely rare for a patient to come for treatment with something other than an obvious physical condition. These days, it is the 'norm' for a patient to attend suffering from stress-related and mental conditions. There are some wonderful acupoints and reflexes that can be used to aid self-healing in emotional imbalance.

Stress has been defined as the specific response of a body to any demand. Stress represents a stimulus or force that produces a reaction. Stress is any life experience that causes physical, mental and emotional change in the individual that results in a state of internal imbalance. It can be physical, such as an injury or exposure to temperature extremes or toxic materials; or psychological, such as the emotional response of anxiety, depression, anger, guilt or hurt engendered by a potential threat; it can even be pleasure derived from an exciting experience. The stress experienced depends not upon the agent that produces it, but upon the person involved and the way he or she reacts.

The 'triad' link between physical, emotional and chemical has been known and accepted within traditional medicine for centuries (see Figure 2.1). It is comparatively recently that medical research has proved the link between stress and emotion and ensuing physical symptoms. There is no doubt in my mind that a large proportion of so-called physical conditions have an emotional aetiology – therefore if emotional imbalance can be treated at an early stage of development, many organic conditions can be prevented. My own research over the past few years has shown me that there is a huge psychosomatic influence in many more physical conditions that hitherto was thought to be the case. Each internal organ, muscle group, vertebral level and joint is related to an emotion in the possible imbalance of that system. This topic is too large to cover in this chapter, but data is being collected for a book on the subject, including treatment and balancing with acupressure and reflextherapy. It is appreciated that innumerable books have been published on the whole topic of psychoneuroimmunology and how the immune system is affected by psycho/emotional states, but nothing has been published on the treatment of these conditions by touch therapy.

Traditional Chinese medicine (TCM) states that there is a correlation between meridians and generalized emotional imbalance. This knowledge can often be used as a starting point in the diagnosis and assessment of emotional imbalance. It may also be used as part of the treatment schedule. The correlations are as follows:

Lung meridian

It is said that prolonged grief and sadness causes energy imbalance in the lung meridian, and to a certain extent, its Yang counterpart – large intestine. Prolonged grief and sadness deplete lung Chi and may manifest in a variety of symptoms, such as breathlessness, tiredness, depression, crying a lot and immune system depletion.

Large intestine

As stated above, prolonged grief and sadness may affect the large intestine meridian. It gives rise to symptoms such as irritable bowel syndrome and diarrhoea. The large intestine meridian energy is, however, mostly affected by lack of expression and the inability to express emotions. When people 'bottle things up' and dwell on life events without having the outlet of counseling or a receptive ear, the large intestine is often the first organ to be affected. Symptoms here would be constipation, bloating, flatulence and abdominal pain. There may also be some mild skin symptoms such as erythema or eczema. Prolonged states of 'lack of emotional freedom' may give symptoms along the course of the large intestine meridian, giving stiff neck, frozen shoulder, sore elbow and generalized joint stiffness.

Stomach

The main mental counterpart of the stomach meridian is worry. Prolonged worry causes stomach Chi depletion, giving symptoms such as acid indigestion, heartburn and stomach ulcers. If the worry becomes prolonged, it could manifest itself as depression, which also affects stomach Chi.

Spleen

Whereas the stomach meridian is affected by worries in general, the spleen is affected by worry and pensiveness by excessive mental work or study. When the spleen is affected, it can cause immune system deficiency, tiredness, loss of appetite and loose stools.

Liver

Liver energy imbalance is traditionally associated with anger. The very broad term of anger may be broken down into other emotions that also affect the liver. These are resentment, repressed anger, irritability, frustration, rage, indignation, animosity or bitterness. Any of these emotional states can affect the liver if they persist for a long time, causing stagnation of liver Chi or rising of liver Yang. Typical symptoms would be headaches, migraine, dizziness, red face and neck and hypertension. Diarrhoea may also ensue, as may muscle tension. Depression may also occur from a long-standing liver Chi imbalance.

Gall bladder

Because of the close ties between the liver and gall bladder, all the emotional imbalances attributed to liver imbalance also affect the gall bladder. The gall bladder is specifically affected in the area of prolonged bitterness and envy. This may give rise to hemi-cranial headaches, stomach upsets and biliousness. If these resentments are not treated correctly, calculii may form in the gall bladder, which in turn causes colic, sickness and vomiting.

Kidney

This meridian is associated with fear. Fear depletes kidney Chi. In his book *The Foundations of Chinese Medicine*, Giovanni Maciocia states

> … in my opinion, fear has a different effect in children and adults. In children, it makes Chi descend causing nocturnal enuresis (bed-wetting). This common problem in children is often caused by fear or a feeling of insecurity in the child due to some family situation. In adults, however, fear and chronic anxiety often cause deficiency of kidney Yin and rising of Empty-Heat within the Heart, with a feeling of heat in the face, night sweating, palpitations and a dry mouth and throat.

Fear is the most common and most primeval of all emotions. Because of its 'ancestral' quality, it affects the kidney energy more than any other organ and meridian. Fear of a prolonged nature also affects the adrenal glands causing adrenal overload, high cortisol levels and subsequent symptoms of nervousness and anxiety. It is, therefore, kidney energy that is mostly affected in long-term emotional conditions. This can give rise to such diverse symptoms as joint stiffness, prostatitis, weak spines, hypertension and cardiac imbalance.

Bladder

The bladder has, obviously, a great affinity with the kidney, therefore it too is involved in many of the same emotions. The simplest example of this is when anxiety causes much 'penny spending'. Another long-term effect of fear is to have problems with the spine – stiffness, laxity or scoliosis. Stiffness occurs when there is combined fear and anxiety; laxity occurs with long-term fear and eating disorders (stomach, spleen and gall bladder energies affect the tendons and soft tissues); scoliosis can occur with the preceding two factors plus the genetic predisposition for it to happen. Turning this on its head and knowing the amazing interaction of body and mind, it is possible that a long-term scoliosis in a person may predispose a nervous breakdown or fear and anxiety. This is generally because the sympathetic nervous system is put under a lot of strain in a curved spine.

Small intestine

This organ/meridian is associated with assimilation. Physical symptoms may occur in people who suffer from long-term indecision. Many people cannot make decisions or make up their minds over even trifling matters. A weakness here may give rise to small bowel symptoms of bloating, abdominal pain and ileo-caecal valve syndrome. The small intestine may also be affected by prolonged sadness.

Heart

Heart energy is traditionally associated with excess joy. Joy is obviously a positive emotion and should create relaxation and engender good health. Joy makes the mind peaceful and relaxed, it benefits the nutritive and defensive Chi and makes Chi relax and slow down. Excess joy is obviously not a healthy contentment but one of excessive excitement that can injure the heart. Over excitement and over-stimulation of the mind can lead to heart fire that can give symptoms such as agitation, insomnia and palpitations. The heart is also said to control the person's spirituality, and that diffidence to one's beliefs may cause imbalance within the heart. Heart energy is also associated with overwork and stress. Too much work may result in depletion of heart Chi, which may give rise to symptoms of angina pectoris or other acute cardiac imbalance.

There are no traditional emotional associations of either the pericardium or three heater meridians, although points on both channels are extensively used in the treatment of emotional conditions.

All the above symptoms that emanate from meridian imbalance may all be improved with good healthy eating, plenty of recreation time and exercise as well as acupressure. Do not forget that these conditions should not be treated in isolation without reference to other forms of natural healing.

Assessment

The assessment in stress, emotional and mental conditions is exactly the same as for organic and physical conditions – why should there be any difference? Following observation of the patient, listening to their story and the usual palpation areas the important part of analysis lies in the listening posts. The main listening post areas are the cranial base, individual cranial points and the heel. It is an individual choice as to which area should be used. The criteria that I have followed are detailed below.

The cranial base or vault hold should be used with any patient who is suffering any degree of stress. The contraindications are in those people who suffer from head clonus (shaking) from a neurological condition or aging. It is impossible to keep the head still in order to concentrate sufficiently. Some patients do not like having their heads touched, this may stem from a physical abuse in their childhood or because they suffer from chronic headaches or psoriasis on the head. Generally though, it remains a very comforting procedure for the majority of patients. The procedure follows that as outlined in treatment of physical conditions, but the emphasis here is to attempt to reach the root cause of the emotional imbalance. It may be emotional trauma, physical injury, abuse or one of a hundred other causes. Questions are asked of the body about the cause. This sometimes requires the patient to assist the therapist by answering out loud any questions that are obscure or have not been asked during the interview. For example, a patient may request treatment for anxiety. Silent questions will be asked by the practitioner as to the organic and physical state of the patient before attempting to ascertain if there is an emotional cause (always ask the obvious first). Questions should then be asked about the patient's birth (possible trauma), childhood, relationships, lifestyle changes, workload etc. The cranial rhythm will change when there is a positive reply. It is quite possible for the patient to 'pick up' on what is happening to them and they may become emotional. This is perfectly OK. It is good to have an emotional response. Be ready with the tissues. Many a patient has been 'cured' during the assessment without the need for actual treatment!

The individual points on the cranium used in emotional imbalance are GB 14 and Si 19. Please refer to Figure 2.19 for their locations. GB 14 should be used whenever the exciting cause of the present symptoms is known, and the patient is sufficiently motivated and willing to be able to express their feelings about the cause. If the patient tells you that they have not been well since a particular episode in their lives, which has obvious important emotional significance to them, this point should be used. It is said to be the 'hypnotherapy point'. Please be aware that the procedure should only be used by experienced practitioners and only with carefully selected clients. With the patient lying down, the therapist should position him or herself at their heads and gently place the middle finger pads on each GB 14 point. Make sure that the arms are well supported as these points may be held for up to 10 minutes. The points should be held for about 1 minute until there is adequate energy feedback before questioning can commence. Do not be in a hurry to commence questioning; there has to be a good energy link between the therapist and the patient. Now ask the patient to think hard about their present symptoms and let them dwell on this for a few seconds. Now ask them to imagine what lies under these symptoms, and what picture comes to mind. They dwell with this picture for about 10 seconds before proceeding to the next layer, and so on. The patient is permitted to speak out loud but the procedure is best done with just thought and visualizing. When they arrive at an episode of their lives that holds the root cause of their present symptoms, there will be a change in their breathing pattern and/or posture. They often will take a huge breath or the breathing may become smoother. They may well express themselves emotionally, so be handy with the tissues. As the reader can see, this point represents an excellent analysis and treatment point in all cases where psychotherapy would normally be the first treatment of choice. I have used this technique thousands of times and had amazing results. Patients may also be instructed to use these two points themselves, but arms tend to ache in self-treatment, so lots of cushions are required to support the arms.

Si 19 is used when there is much tension and stress, especially in the TMJ (temporo-mandibular joint or jaw joint). TMJs are often affected by stress, so much so that it is sometimes difficult for affected people to open their mouths sufficiently to speak or eat properly. This is obviously a worst-case scenario, but I have witnessed this three or four times. The TMJ becomes tight and in spasm due to a number of factors. There is often a history of bad dentistry or an old accident or injury that has affected the lower jaw, thus causing mal-alignment. People who grind their teeth at night may also have TMJ spasm. Another cause could be energy imbalance within the small intestine, gall bladder or heating mechanism, as these are the meridians that are adjacent to the joint. As with the treatment of GB 14, the therapist holds the pads of the middle fingers on Si 19 for about a minute, until heat and energy can be felt under the fingers. This hold may be used for assessment in ascertaining the cause of the TMJ tension, or it could be used for treatment in order to slowly ease the spasm and pain. This may not occur in the first treatment session, but even long term pain and spasm should release in time. If the cause of the TMJ discomfort is ascertained, the treatment, by acupressure, can then commence – see page 103 of *Acupressure: Clinical Applications in Musculo-skeletal Conditions*.

The heel is an excellent listening post, especially when the therapist is dealing with emotional and mental health. It should be used in all cases where patients do not like having their head held, in babies and children, as an overture to using foot reflexology and with patients who may be aggressive or mentally unbalanced. A physiotherapist who attended one of my workshops cited her work in prison hospitals. She said that even though she had the luxury of having a chaperone with her, she felt much safer to work with the feet as opposed to the head in initial encounters with patients. She could then transfer to the head, and other parts of the body when she had gained the patient's confidence, and indeed, the patient felt more comfortable in her company and her way of doing things. The therapist should position themselves at the patient's feet with them lying down or in long sitting. With the forearms supported on the couch, both heels are held and 'cuddled', i.e. their left heel in the right hand and the right heel in the left hand. The heels should be held for about 2 minutes before any further work is attempted. There *has* to be a feeling of oneness with the patient and the therapist, otherwise very little will happen. After about 2 minutes has elapsed, try and pick up the Chi flow within the body. This is done by sensing a gentle expansion and contraction under the heels. When this has been felt, try and expand this sensation under the hands to create a 'balloon' effect of energy. This inward and outward motion that has been created is exactly the same as tuning in to the cerebrospinal fluid (CSF) flow in the cranial base. To use this technique in analysis, questions are asked as before. When the answers to the questions are negative, the flow remains; when the answer is positive, the flow ceases. Questions can be tuned finer and finer so as to come to an exact diagnosis or analysis. This technique may also be used in treatment mode. The first stage is to project Chi (by thought) up the legs and into the body when there is maximum expansion of Chi under the hands. This affords amazing relaxation in the patient and if done over a period of about 10 minutes can be enough treatment in its own right. The second stage if required, is to project Chi (by thought) to specific areas of the body that need to be energy balanced. This whole routine is the overture to a specific type of reflexology that has been coined light touch reflexology. Further details on this whole topic will be in the next publication.

Treatment of named conditions

As has been mentioned before, the treatment of these conditions does not differ from the treatment of other medical conditions. The exception is that there is no need to massage the Chapman's reflexes. The batting order of treatment is therefore:

1. Stroke the associated meridian.
2. Stimulate the associated great point.
3. Stimulate and energy balance the related special points.
4. Stimulate the energy point.
5. Balance the general energy via the Sheng cycle. This is either Yin or Yang depending on the condition.

Anxiety and nervousness

Definition: A neurotic disorder characterized by chronic, unrealistic emotional stress often punctuated by acute attacks of anxiety or panic.

Emotional stress often precipitates anxiety (e.g. threatened or actual changes in personal relationships). Anxiety represents the individual's fear of losing control and of the resultant reactions. The symptoms of anxiety are the direct manifestations of the peripheral nervous system discharge (fight or flight reactions) set in motion by the arousal of frightening fantasies, impulses and emotions. In the central nervous system, noradrenergic neurotransmitters play a prominent role in the production of anxiety. Recent studies point to the locus ceruleus, with its widespread connecting neural pathways to the rest of the brain, as an important mediating centre. Anxiety is a symptom in most stress, emotional and mental disorders, but it occurs alone in anxiety neurosis and chronic nervousness. Acute anxiety attacks (panic disorders) form the cardinal feature of anxiety neurosis and are among the most painful of all life experiences. They are more common in women and tend to die out in middle age. Naturopathically, anxiety and nervousness arises when a person does not trust the flow and the process of life. The worry, inability to relax, fear, insomnia, tension or lack of confidence are caused by any emotional trauma or happening, conditioning or belief system due to lack of faith.

Treatment with acupressure and reflextherapy (Figure 6.1)

Acute panic attacks, as previously explained, are awful experiences for the sufferers, and those who are fortunate enough not to know what it is like, simply have no idea of the torment and anguish that occurs. The worst thing that someone else can do is to tell the person to 'snap out of it'. They should be reassured and brought gently out of the situation that is causing the panic. This may be impossible if the attack occurs in an airplane or in

Figure 6.1 Points used in anxiety and nervousness.

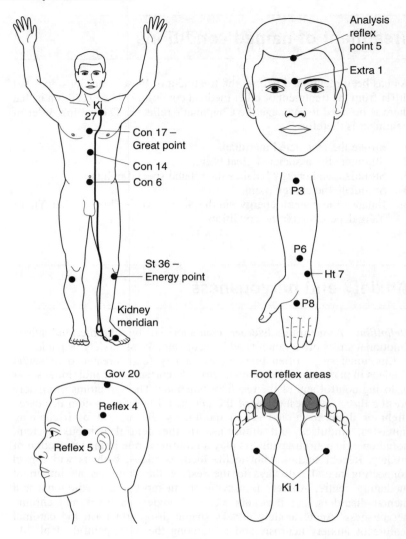

the middle of a crowded theatre. The person should be encouraged to take deep breaths, dwelling longer on the expiration than the inspiration. They should also be encouraged to stimulate Con 17, which is located in the middle of the sternum. This is the great point for anxiety, acute or chronic. Reassurance is the key to dealing with panic. The sufferer must be told that they are in control, that they are not suffering a heart attack, going mad or going to die (as they often feel all these things), but that the symptoms they are having are inflammation of the sympathetic nervous system in response to their situation.

Treatment of chronic anxiety and nervousness by a therapist

1. The associated meridian is the kidney channel. This is indicated because the root psychological cause of anxiety and nervousness is

fear. It is often the case that the patient has no idea where the fear comes from, but by stroking the kidney channel 10 times in the direction of energy flow, this should make inroads into creating relaxation and easing tension in the adrenals.

2. The great point is Con 17, located in the centre of the sternum at the level of the nipples. It is always a tender point when it needs treatment. The patient should be relaxed in the supine lying position and the point should be stimulated for about 4 minutes. During this time, the patient should start to sigh and take deep gulps of breath in response to the treatment. Con 17 is specific for easing tension and feelings of constriction in the chest. In severe and acute anxiety, the first point that should be used is Ki 1. This is a really magical point when used correctly. Position yourself at the patient's feet and gently touch bilateral Ki 1 with the finger pads of the middle fingers. After about 2 minutes of just touching the point (do not stimulate) a change of emphasis should be felt. It will be at this point that the patient should start to feel more relaxed. This point may be held for a further couple of minutes or so, or Con 17 can now be stimulated. An even more effective way of using Ki 1 in acute neurosis is by taking the fingers about half an inch away from the foot and keeping them still above the point. The effect is more powerful than touching the body. Using the first part of the etheric body is often more powerful than touching the skin. This aspect of healing will be fully covered in the next book in the series.

3. There are several special points that the therapist may use to supplement the effect of Con 17. Each has a slightly different action, so not all points will be needed. They are located on the scalp, chest and abdomen, arm and foot.

Scalp points

*   Gov 20, located at the crown of the head, traditionally called the point of a thousand meetings, is the ideal point for calming the whole body, physical and emotional. It is said to be the meeting point of all the Yang channels and clears all excess Yang energy in the head. It clears the mind and lifts the spirits. It is a good point for clearing brain fog and heaviness. There is a contraindication though – do not stimulate it when there is hypertension. Ideally, as mentioned in a previous chapter, placing both hands on the scalp and easing the fingers apart should gently stretch the point.

*   Reflex point 5 is located on the Pterion where the greater wing of the sphenoid bone can be felt. It is said to have a direct access to the hypothalamus, hence its role in calming the sympathetic nervous system and clearing brain fog. It is also an excellent point for lowering hypertension in anxiety. The procedure is to place the middle finger pads of both hands on each point and gently, slowly give a little stimulation for a minute or so, before keeping the fingers still for a further 2 minutes. The results can be amazing.

*   Reflex point 4, located 1 cun above the ear, in the temple, is a very good point for relaxing the mind from extraneous thoughts and for general calming.

*   Extra 1 (Gov 24.5) is the anterior equivalent of the brow Chakra and is one of the best points there is for relaxing the mind and allaying anxiety. It may be used in isolation or in combination with Gov 16. When using this point as self-treatment, it is important that the head is supported on a pillow. Also support the

arm with a pillow on the side of the head so the arm doesn't tire. Try an energy balance between this point and Con 17, it is very powerful.

- Reflex point 11 is a superb point used in the treatment of anxiety. This point, illustrated in Figure 3.16, is located in the centre line just below the hairline. It can be used in analysis (see Figure 3.17, where it is called point 5) or as treatment. It is the very best point to use in accessing the autonomic nervous system. In the treatment of anxiety and nervousness, it should never be stimulated. It should be held gently for up to 5 minutes or until a change of emphasis is felt, when an amazing relaxation of the whole system will be felt. The practitioner should be aware of the power in this point; it can easily make someone relax enough so as to go to sleep.

Chest and abdomen points

- Ki 27, located in the depression between the first rib and the lower border of the clavicle, 2 cun lateral from the midline, eases tension in the chest and neck that may be caused by anxiety. It may also be stimulated to address an imbalance within the thyroid gland, which often occurs in anxiety and nervousness. The point should be sedated, no stimulated and the energy balanced with Con 17.

- Con 14 is located just below the xiphoid sternum. It is said to be the physical counterpart of the anterior solar plexus chakra, and as such, is a powerful point in the treatment of many psychological conditions, including anxiety. It calms the mind, eases angina, treats excess stomach energy caused by emotional turmoil and helps disperse excess energy within the solar (coeliac) plexus of the autonomic nervous system. It is also said to be the pivotal point along the conception channel and is important in creating equilibrium between energies above (thorax) and below (abdomen). It is therefore an excellent balancing point where the patient complains of heat in the top of the body and cold in the bottom, or heat along the front and cold on the back.

- Con 6 is located 1.5 cun below the umbilicus. It is a very powerful acupoint and has many properties. It is said to be the Hara point and is extensively used in meditation, yoga and pranic breathing. When stimulated, it is used for lethargy and tiredness, both physical and mental. Chronic anxiety and nervousness can create an enormous amount of fatigue in the body attempting to stabilize energy all the time – being ill is exhausting! It has many other local effects in easing tension in the abdomen, bladder and vagina and also in dealing with fluid retention in the abdomen and ankles. It is a very useful point in treating chronic psychosomatic conditions.

Arm points

- P 3 is located in the middle of the transverse cubital crease on the ulnar side of the biceps tendon. It is said to be the water point of the pericardium channel, and as such, calms down the fire within the meridian and the area of the body that it supplies. It tends to pacify the stomach and heart and is excellent in easing the pain of angina or the chest pains that often accompany anxiety – many a panic attack has seemed like a heart attack. It is a very good point in calming the mind and in cases of severe anxiety with chest or thoracic spinal pain. The energy balance between P 3 and Con 17 is a particularly effective one.

- P 6 is one of the fundamental points in acupuncture and acupressure with a number of different functions. It has already been described in earlier chapters as one of the most useful points in the treatment of nausea, lethargy, and menstrual and endocrine imbalance. It also has a powerful calming action on the mind and can be used in anxiety caused by overwork, stress, food intolerance and worry. It may also be used for irritability and anger, along with liver points.
- P 8 is located in the centre of the palm. It is said to be the hand chakra with direct esoteric links with the foot chakra at Ki 1 and the crown chakra at Gov 20. It is this triad of points that is very effective in balancing the body's general energy system in chronic anxiety. P 8 remains one of the unsung heroes in acupressure. It has already been described as a useful point in hypertension, but its greatest claim to fame is in calming the mind. It seems to be the most effective point in clearing heart-fire and for producing relaxation in the upper body. Try balancing it with Con 17 and then balance it with Ki 1 and Gov 20. You will be surprised by the influential results.
- Ht 7, located on the radial side of the anterior wrist crease, has already been described as the great point of the heart meridian and one of the very best points in insomnia. The TCM word for this point is *Shenmen*, which means 'Spirit Gate' or 'Mind Door'. It is therefore the most useful point in the treatment of acute anxiety next to Con 17. It may also be used in poor memory and stress due to worry. Giovanni Maciocia, in his book *The Foundations of Chinese Medicine* says of this point, 'As the Heart is the residence for the Mind, which in Chinese Medicine includes mental activity, thinking, memory and consciousness, this point has an effect not only on emotional problems such as anxiety, but also on memory and mental capacity. In fact, this point can be used for mental retardation in children'. There is also a Shenmen point in the ear that is used in poor memory and concentration.

Foot points
- Ki 1 has already been described as the point of choice in the first instance in treating extreme anxiety and restlessness. It is extremely useful in clearing 'brain fog' and headaches due to stress and tension. It can be used in isolation or balancing it with P 8 and Gov 20. The logistical problems of balancing the sole of the foot with the top of the head can be overcome with the patient in long sitting with their knees bent up.
- Finally, but not least, the reflex areas on the foot that represent the head can be most influential in the balancing of anxiety and nervousness. I would use this reflex every time in the treatment of chronic anxiety states. Although the area of the great toe is shown in Figure 6.1, this is only a representation of what can be treated on the foot to ease the nervous system. In general reflexology practice, the central nervous system reflexes should always be massaged first to balance perceptions and encourage the appropriate physical, emotional and spiritual responses. Brain reflexes are found on the pads and nails of all the toes, cerebral reflexes on the tips and cervical reflexes on the base of each toe. Midbrain reflexes are found along the inner edge of the great toes. All these areas should be gently stimulated as part of the whole

treatment. Please do not apply a great deal of pressure on these reflexes, there is far better reaction when they are used gently.

4. The energy point for this condition is St 36. This point should be stimulated for up to 2 minutes following the main treatment session. Care must be taken in stimulating this point if the patient has just eaten or is suffering from nausea or upset stomach.

5. The body's general energy system should now be balanced via the Sheng cycle of the five elements circle. The Yang circle should be used in children and when the condition is acute, and the Yin cycle should be used in all chronic conditions (see Figures 4.1 and 5.1).

Non-acupressure treatment

To have a healthy mind, the same advice is given as for those who are striving to have a healthy body – there is no difference. Eat plenty of nutritious food and avoid too much protein, red meat, dairy produce, sugar and preservatives. The following herbs and homoeopathic remedies are recommended for anxiety:

(a) Kava kava is derived from the root of the Australian shrub, *Piper methysticum*. It helps reduce anxiety, aid restful sleep and also is of use during the menopause. It is taken ideally at the end of the day to unwind from the stresses and strains of the day.

(b) Valerian should be taken more for insomnia than anxiety, but as many patients who suffer from anxiety also have insomnia, it is recommended that it is take just before sleeping. It is the main ingredient in many of the proprietary brand herbal sleeping remedies.

(c) The best homoeopathic remedy for anxiety is aconite, which is derived from monkshood. It is a specific remedy for anxiety, restlessness and fright. The 30th potency is probably the most effective and should be taken at 15-minute intervals until the symptoms subside (try giving it to a child who wakes up in the small hours screaming with earache, sore throat or fever – it works a treat; it is just like turning off a tap!).

Depression

Definition: Depression is a psychopathological mood disorder, which is either a primary determinant or constitutes the core manifestation. Depression may be acute or chronic and have many causes. There are various types of depression and most people experience a degree of depression at some stage of their lives. Reactive depression is a response to a particular emotional trauma; neurotic depression is a reaction to the misfortunes encountered; endogenous depression has no specific cause but often follows a viral infection, hormonal changes after childbirth etc. Symptoms may be fatigue, insomnia, weakness, no drive, weeping, sadness, lack of interest, despair and aches and pains. Clinical depression is usually treated with psychotherapy or anti-depressive drugs of various kinds. Research has shown, though, that when either of these treatments is combined with exercise therapy, the results obtained are improved. Depression rarely exists alone, in that a prospective patient who is suffering from depression is not likely to consult a 'hands-on' therapist unless there are other over-riding physical symptoms. It often occurs that the root cause of the depression will present itself when taking the case sheet or during treatment. Where an overriding mood disorder presents itself, it is essential that this syndrome be treated first, almost at the expense of treating any physical condition. This obeys the naturopathic laws of treatment that states that the spiritual overrides the emotional /mental that in turn overrides the physical. If the mental condition is treated successfully, very many of the physical symptoms will also be alleviated. The only possible exception to this is that if the physical sensation of pain is eased, the spirits are raised and the mental condition should be eased somewhat. Whatever type of depression or symptoms the patient is suffering from, the one thing that someone should never do is to ask them to 'snap out of it'. They would if they could! Having said this, many types of depression are purely self-induced, and if patients can be shown where the cause lies, it is very possible that they can reverse the cause of the disease.

Treatment by acupressure and reflextherapy (Figure 6.2)

1. The associated meridian is the stomach channel. Traditional Chinese medicine states that the stomach is the seat of depressive illness. What is meant by this is not altogether clear, but two theories spring to mind. Firstly, the stomach represents the centre and 'earth' of a person, indeed it is an organ belonging to the Earth element. It represents the mid-way junction between Heaven and Man, at the solar plexus, and is therefore a pivotal organ and energy system and is responsible for filtering esoteric energies between one and the other. This aspect of esoteric medicine will be full discussed in the next book. Secondly, it has been shown that faulty eating can both cause and prolong depression. Depression can result from over eating sugars and other complicated carbohydrates. The stomach meridian should be stroked up to 10 times in the direction of energy flow – from the head towards the second toe. This can be performed through clothes but concentration of effort should be made at the lower end of the meridian between the knee and foot. One word of practical advice in the treatment of women – as the stomach meridian passes over the breast (the nipple is St 17), make sure that the patient is fully aware of what is about to happen before the stroking commences. If in doubt, make sure that a chaperone is with you!

2. The great point in this condition is St 36. What an amazingly versatile point this is. By stimulating this point on a regular basis it will increase the body's general energy, increase stomach and spleen energy and help stabilize the 'Earth' of the patient. This point should be stimulated for about 3 minutes before proceeding onto the next part of the session. Do not over-stimulate this point if the patient is suffering from nausea or stomach upset.

3. There are 11 special points that can be used to supplement St 36. I have purposely not included reflex points with this condition. It isn't because they are ineffective – on the contrary, they are superb – but there are no individual points that stand out. Instead the best way to

Figure 6.2 Points used in depression.

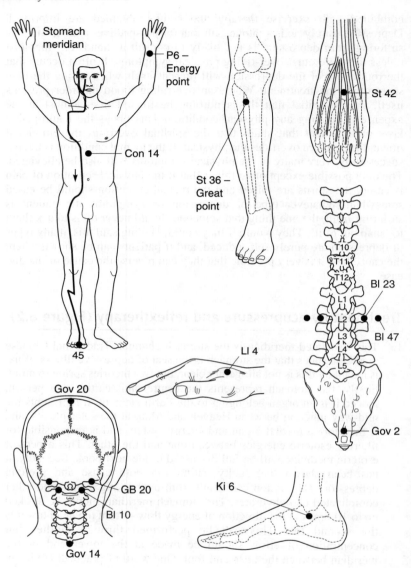

treat purely with reflextherapy is to do a full foot reflex pattern and treat the patient holistically – it works wonders.

- Gov 20 has been discussed in the treatment of anxiety. It is also an excellent point in depressive illness in that it raises the spirits. The point should be *gently* stimulated for up to a minute and then just held and balanced with St 36. This is a wonderful balance and the patient will start to feel much easier following it. Gov 20 may also be treated by a 'hands-off' approach. Leave the whole of the hand, centred about a centimetre above the crown of the head, for about 2 minutes. This can be done in isolation or it can be balanced with St 36 (this point is touched).
- LI 4 has a reputation in alleviating pain and discomfort in the head and neck region. Depression sometimes gives physical symptoms of

brain fog, dizziness and fullness, and LI 4 is an excellent point in relieving these symptoms. The point also clears the mind and eases tension, especially in people who have the dreaded combination of depression and anxiety.

- GB 20, Bl 10 and Gov 14 are used to clear the head, ease tension in the neck and cranial base muscles, ease discomfort, improve energy and ease irritability. Gov 14 is particularly useful in easing tension at the back of the head and neck, which often accompanies depression. Gov 14 is also the posterior aspect of the throat chakra. Stimulating this point helps in giving energy to the thyroid gland, thus improving the body's general energy levels; also it clears the mind and allows self-expression to take place. I have witnessed this on innumerable occasions. It tends to 'loosen the tongue' in patients who have difficulty expressing themselves. Depression is always eased when sufferers are allowed to talk freely (a trouble shared is a trouble halved). Gov 14 may be used in isolation or in combination with the anterior throat chakra point – Con 22.

- Bl 23 and Bl 47, located at the level of L2–L3, are used to treat the effects of tiredness and lethargy in that they stimulate adrenal and cortisol production. They should be stimulated for about 4 minutes in order to be effective. Patients with confirmed disc protrusions should be careful when stimulating these points. Patients should be encouraged to use these points in self-treatment. They should be rubbed with the medial border of the clenched fist for at least 2 minutes, four times per day.

- Ki 6 is located just inferior to the medial malleolus. It tends to calm the mind and increase kidney energy, thus helping to overcome the fear that may be one of the causes of the depression. Try balancing Ki 6 with St 36 after both points have been stimulated for about 1 minute. It is amazing how well this procedure boosts energy and helps clear the mind.

- St 42 is located on the highest part of the dorsum of the foot. This point represents a treasure trove in acupressure. If it is used in acupuncture, there seem to be limited indications such as local foot pain and toothache. When it is stimulated with acupressure it seems to be the best point on the lower stomach meridian to help boost stomach energy, thus helping boost stomach Yin and subsequently helping with depression. This point works best if the cause of the depression is one of faulty eating over several years.

- The final special point is Gov 2. This point is located in the midline between the sacrum and coccyx. Its anatomical positioning often puts practitioners off using it more. It is the posterior aspect of the base chakra and should be used to treat *any* chronic condition, especially if there is a familial taint, i.e. depression appears in the immediate family. This point, of any other in the body, is the best one for boosting energy in chronic conditions. It should be stimulated for about 4–5 minutes in the treatment session, with the patient lying prone. It can be performed with the patient clothed so as to offset embarrassment. After about 2 minutes of stimulation, the patient will feel warmth down the legs, followed shortly by warmth and a feeling of 'lightness' up the spine.

4. The energy point in this condition is P 6. It should be stimulated for a couple of minutes following the main treatment. This helps boost and maintain the energy that has been induced in the treatment.

5. Finally, the general energy should be balanced by using the Yin circle of the Sheng cycle.

Non-acupressure treatment

Mention has already been made of eating correctly. Patients should be encouraged to eat simple sugars (fructose and glucose) and cut out complex carbohydrates. They should also eat lots of vegetables and pulses. They should also be encouraged, at all costs, to stop smoking. As with the treatment of anxiety, there are several herbal and homoeopathic remedies that can be tried as an alternative to anti-depressant remedies. Vitamin C, with added bioflavin, should be taken daily. It is recommended that 1 g a day is taken in two tablets of 500 mg, morning and evening. St John's wort has had a huge press in the last few years as being helpful in mild depression. It is undoubtedly true that anecdotal evidence tends to suggest that it is helpful in many people. Some sufferers, though, find that it does absolutely nothing to help their symptoms. It is possible that the dosage is incorrect. It is recommended that at least 900 µg of hypercin, the active ingredient, is taken daily. I was astonished when St John's wort came to prominence as an anti-depressive remedy. I had always used it either as a tincture or as a low potency homoeopathic remedy (Hypericum) as a remedy to treat nerve pain. On the subject of homoeopathic remedies, the best remedy to ease acute and mild depression is Ignatia 6, taken four times a day. The best remedy for easing chronic depression symptoms is Arg. Nit 30, taken twice a day. There is no substitute, however, for consulting a qualified homoeopathic practitioner who can work out the correct constitutional remedy for the patient.

Irritability and anger

Irritability is defined as an irrational behavioural pattern manifesting itself in anger, bad temper, irrationality and diffidence. It is the reaction, borne out of frustration, of an event or series of events occurring in one's life. It may be acute or chronic. Acute anger and irritability is sometimes a healthy reaction to stress. Psychologists are always stressing the importance of letting go of the emotions and not bottling anger up. It is when these frustrations in life's pattern are bottled up and suppressed that energy and subsequent organic changes may occur. Whereas prolonged anxiety can affect the kidney and prolonged depression can affect the stomach and the immune system, so prolonged anger and frustration can affect the liver. Symptoms include muscle spasm, headaches and migraine, dizziness, hypertension, lethargy and hyperactivity.

Treatment by acupressure and reflextherapy (Figure 6.3)

1. The associated meridian is the liver channel. This should be stroked up to a dozen times bilaterally with special emphasis around the foot to

Figure 6.3 Points used in depression.

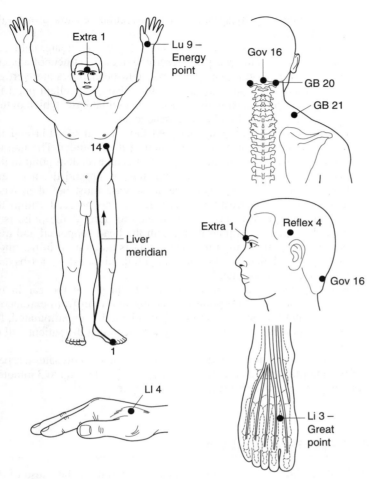

the knee. It should be stroked in the direction of energy flow in chronic conditions and against the flow in acute flare-ups

2. The great point in irritability and anger is Li 3. Li 3 is the source point of the liver and consequently has a direct influence on the organ. The point should be stimulated in all cases of stress and irritability for up to 3 minutes. If this is performed in tandem with LI 4, the benefit to the patient is increased. Li 3 is the most prominent point on the liver channel for subduing liver Yang which always gives rise to headaches, muscle aches and liver toxicity. It is also useful in the treatment of muscle cramp and eyestrain.

3. There are seven special points that can be used to support the effect of Li 3.

    • LI 4 has already been mentioned as the main accompanying point to Li 3. It is the ideal overture of a treatment session. The two points should be stimulated for a couple of minutes and then just held and energy balanced for a further 2 minutes or until a change of emphasis is noted. Make sure your patient does not go to sleep before feeling pleasures in store with the remainder of the session! LI 4 may be used in isolation when there is eyestrain, headache, sinus congestion, hypertension and muscular tension around the head and neck.

- Balancing Extra 1 (Gov 24.5) and Gov 16 together creates calm and clears the mind. This was fully described in the treatment of anxiety.
- GB 20 is used to eliminate dizziness, light-headedness and vertigo, which often accompany irritability. It is also an excellent point for treating muscular tension in the neck and cranial base, which in turn often clears occipital and frontal headaches.
- GB 21 is located midway between Gov 14 (at C7–T1) and the acromium process at the highest point of the shoulder. The first rib should be palpable beneath this point. It is an excellent point in this syndrome as it helps ease muscular tension around the neck and head. It can be a very tender point, so care must be taken when approaching it for treatment, start gently and proceed within the patient's tolerance levels. The best way to 'attack' the point is to have the patient in supine lying, with the head supported and treat both points at the same time. This point is much used in treatment of musculo-skeletal conditions including elevated first ribs and thoracic inlet syndrome.
- Reflex point 4 on the head, located 1 cun above the ear in the temple, is a very good point in relaxing the mind from extraneous thought and for general calming. It can be held, not stimulated, for up to 5 minutes, when it is almost guaranteed that the patient will be asleep.

4. The energy point in this condition is Lu 9, situated on the lateral aspect of the anterior wrist crease. It should be stimulated for up to 3 minutes.
5. Finally, energy balance using the Sheng cycle.

Non-acupressure treatment

As with all conditions, the ideal treatment is to eliminate the cause of the problem. In the case of chronic irritability and anger, one of the best ways is by consulting a cognitive psychotherapist who will attempt to ascertain the root cause. Food-wise, it is essential that the liver be helped by any means it can. This often means doing a detoxing diet. Sometimes, the object of doing such a diet is defeated because of the ensuing headaches and irritability, but these symptoms will subside when the detoxing is completed. Anecdotal evidence has shown that diet therapy alone has been known to cure very many cases. Herbal remedies that may help would include garlic (to purify and cleanse the system), vitamin C, royal jelly, valerian, magnesium and oil of evening primrose. Homoeopathic remedies that are best suited to people who have this condition would include Nux Vomica 30, taken twice a day until symptoms ease, and Bryonia 6 or 30. Of the two, Bryonia is better suited in acute cases and Nux Vomica in chronic conditions. Yoga, Tai Chi, Chi Gong and meditation will also be of value.

Poor memory and concentration

These syndromes can be very painful experiences. They occur more often in middle age and have few obvious causes. As poor memory prolongs, it can, of course, give rise to senility and many other conditions. There are several predisposing causes. Poor posture through life remains the main culprit. This often produces imbalance in the spinal musculature and ligaments which cause cervical vertebral displacements and cranial imbalance, giving rise to circulatory and lymphatic alterations in the brain. Therefore, it is in the best interest of everyone to adopt a correct posture throughout life so as to prevent repercussions. The second most common cause of poor memory is faulty diet. Eating too much refined sugar puts strain on the stomach, liver and spleen. If this is overdone for decades, there are resultant cellular changes in the liver and pancreas. Chinese medicine tells us that sluggish spleen (pancreas) Chi can affect the memory and concentration as well as mental and emotional stability. Stress over many years can also have a damaging effect on the brain cells. Acupressure treatment can only help mild loss of memory and concentration. It cannot help symptoms of senility.

Treatment with acupressure and reflextherapy (Figure 6.4)

1. There are no associated meridians with these conditions.
2. The great point is Extra 1 (Gov 24.5), located midline between the eyebrows. It is essential in any treatment strategy devised to help a person suffering from poor memory, that they are initially relaxed. The patient is bound to be uptight, stressed and possibly a little embarrassed about their predicament, and they must be put at their ease by starting to relax the mind. The supreme point to do this is Yintang (Extra 1). As the reader is by now aware, this point represents the anterior aspect of the brow (Ajna) chakra. It is therefore used in many ways, but predominantly it has an influence on the pituitary gland. If this point is sedated, there is a knock-on effect of sedation and relaxation in all the other endocrine glands. This has paramount importance in healing. Yintang is a supreme point in acupressure in that it serves to relax the mind and strengthen the will.
3. There are 10 other special points and areas that can be used to augment the use of Yintang.
   - Gov 16. This point is situated in the inion, between the occipital base and the atlas. It is mentioned first because of its special relationship with Yintang. As has already been explained, the two points represent the anterior and posterior aspects of the brow Chakra. They work extremely well in tandem. Traditionally, Yintang is used in Yin conditions and Gov 16 used in Yang conditions, but when used together, they can be used in any condition that warrants their use. It is the supreme duo for inducing relaxation and for clearing the mind from stress, worries and many other emotional disturbances. Patients should be encouraged to use it themselves at regular intervals. The best way for the practitioner

Figure 6.4 Points used in poor memory and concentration.

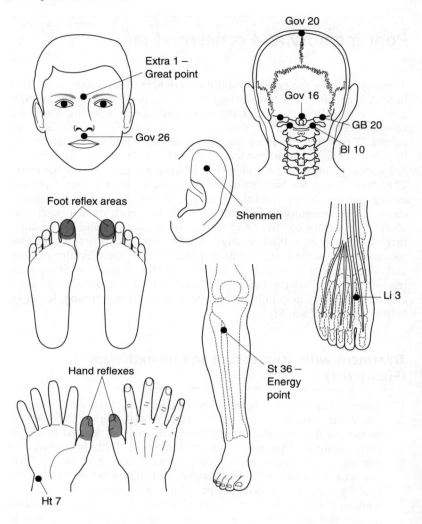

to use the points is to sit comfortably at the head of the patient, who is supine lying with the head supported. Gently introduce the fingers to these two points whilst having the forearms supported. Energy balance between these two can take up to 5 minutes. The following five points may be treated with the therapist and patient in the same mode.

- Gov 20, located at the crown of the head should be initially stimulated for a few seconds before being sedated once the energy has been perceived under the fingers. This point clears the head and mind and lifts the spirits in depression. The energy balance with Yintang is very powerful.
- Gov 26, located two-thirds of the way between the top lip and the nose, has many functions. It has already been mentioned in its role as the anti-sneezing point and also in fainting and dizziness. When the point is stimulated for up to 3 minutes (careful not to mark the patient with the fingernail) it is a very good point for improving the memory and concentration. The patient should be encouraged to use

it daily for 2 minutes each session in conjunction with all the other points that are easily accessible.

- GB 20 and Bl 10, situated at the base of the skull, provide relaxation of the cervical and posterior scalp fascia. They also clear the head and enable 'thinking' to be easier. It is amazing how much tension in the back of the head causes headaches, fullness and fog in the head. These two points are gently stimulated to relieve these symptoms.
- Ht 7, located by the pisiform bone at the medial aspect of the anterior wrist crease, is *the* point to clear a hurried and confused mind. It is a well-known point in the treatment of insomnia. This point should be stimulated with a fair degree of vigour and enthusiasm in order to reap the benefits. The Chinese name for this point is *Shenmen* or *Mind Door*. Shen means 'spirit', and the Chinese thought that the spiritual aspect of health was dealt with via the heart meridian, and Ht 7 in particular. This point, therefore, above every other point on the body is supreme in treating affections of the spirit and mind. It clears the mind and boosts the spiritual energy.
- Shenmen is also to be found as an ear reflex point. The tip of the little finger or a baby bud for up to 2 minutes (no longer) should be used. Some practitioners swear by this point, others would not dream of using it. It is a personal thing.
- Li 3, as has been shown already, is one of the major acupoints in the body that deals with relaxation, clearing the mind, headaches and easing muscular tension and cramping. It has, however, proved to be one of the best points in dealing with poor memory, especially if the cause has been faulty eating over a period of time. The point should be stimulated for about 3 minutes before attempting (with long arms) a balance with Yintang.
- Finally, but in no way least effective are the reflex areas of the foot and hand that correspond with the head, i.e. great toe and thumb. I have already extolled the virtues of the great toe reflexes. The thumb represents a diluted version with regard to its efficacy and power. The patient should, though be encouraged to massage the thumbs as often as possible.

4. The associated energy point in these two syndromes is St 36. This is the master 'energy giving' command point in the body and should be used because of this. St 36 also reinforces Earth Chi, thus giving a stabilizing effect for the patient. It also helps increase the energy and circulatory flow to the head. Do not stimulate this point when the patient is suffering from nausea.
5. Finally, balance the body's general energy system via the Yin aspect of the Sheng cycle.

Non-acupressure treatment

Correct diet has already been mentioned, but it is of paramount importance that the patient adopts a different eating plan to the one that possibly encouraged the condition to commence. It is sometimes extremely difficult for, say, a 70-year-old to radically change their diet, but if they are willing to take advice and stick to it, it will bring enormous rewards. They should be encouraged to take extra lecithin in capsule form as well as concentrating on eating lecithin-rich foods – egg yolk, soya and sweetcorn. Chelated magnesium tablets and ginkgo biloba should also be taken as supplements.

Grief and sadness

Grief and sadness represent two of the emotional states in TCM, which are possible causes of internal disharmony. The others are anger, joy, pensiveness, fear and fright. As mentioned in the chapter's introduction, it is the lung and large intestine that are the organs and meridians most affected. A normal and healthy expression of grief and sadness can be expressed as sobbing that originates in the depths of the lungs – deep breaths and the expulsion of air with the crying. However, sadness that remains unresolved and becomes chronic can create a disharmony in the lungs, making the lung Chi weak. This, in turn, can interfere with the lung's function of circulating Chi around the body. A patient will probably not consult the therapist complaining of sadness or grief. It is the role of the practitioner to ascertain that the root cause of their symptoms is some form of long-term grief or chronic melancholy. Among the symptoms presented would be breathlessness, asthma, tiredness, depression, crying a lot and immune system depletion.

Treatment by acupressure and reflextherapy (Figure 6.5)

1. The associated meridian is, of course, the lung channel. It should be stroked for up to 10 times in the direction of energy flow, i.e. from the chest towards the thumb. Experience has shown that even with this initial treatment, it is possible to cause the patient to show emotion and cry.
2. The great point for this condition is Lu 9. It is located at the lateral aspect of the anterior wrist crease. It is said to be the source point of the lung meridian, hence it affects the lung organ more effectively than any other point. It should be stimulated bilaterally for up to 4 minutes. Other points on the lung channel are also effective, such as Lu 1, Lu 5, Lu 7 and Lu 11. One of the best ways to treat all the points involved is to perform a shiatsu type massage down the meridian. This consists of thumb pad kneading down the channel, dwelling a couple of seconds at each level before moving on to the next one.
3. There are five special points apart from the ones along the course of the lung meridian that may be used to enhance the efficacy of Lu 9 *et al*.
   • Ht 3 is located on the medial aspect of the anterior elbow crease on the same level as Lu 5. Ht 3 is probably the second most powerful point on the heart channel next to Ht 7. It is also ideally situated for self-treatment. It is a very useful point in many emotionally based syndromes and has an important calming action on the mental level.

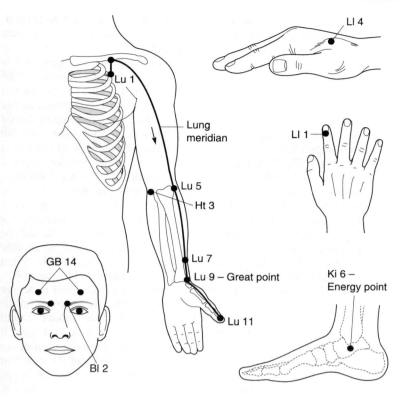

Figure 6.5 Points used in grief and sadness.

It is indicated in epilepsy, depression as well as the symptomatic treatment of sadness and grief. It should be stimulated for about 2 minutes and then energy balanced with Lu 9.

- LI 4 needs no introduction, except to say that it is a wonderful point in the treatment of many emotional conditions. Grief and sadness in the long term give a number of physical symptoms, such as headache, eyestrain, and tightness in the chest etc. that can all be improved by treating LI 4.
- LI 1 is located at the nail point on the lateral aspect of the index finger. It is best known in the treatment of acute toothache of the upper jaw. It remains, though, quite a powerful point in clearing the mind and aiding assimilation of thought processes. Take care not to stimulate it with too much enthusiasm; it can easily become sore and inflamed.
- Bl 2 is located directly above the inner canthus in a small hollow on the medial side of the brow. In acupuncture it is used as a local eye point, and for frontal headache and sinusitis. Acupressure has given this point prominence in utilizing another of its functions. It has been shown that if the point is 'tapped' several times for up to half a minute, it can strengthen the bladder meridian. This, in turn, strengthens the spine and allays fear. It is very important that the spinal muscular system is kept supple and strong in most conditions, but especially in chronic emotional imbalance. There is quite a tie-in between someone who has a weak spine and being a fearful type of person. Stimulating this point by gentle tapping helps to combat

this weakness. This point need not be energy balanced with Lu 9. The patient should be encouraged to tap the point about three times a day for up to half a minute at a time.

- GB 14 is located 1 cun above the midpoint of the eyebrow, and is used in a totally different way to Bl 2. The technique using GB 14 as a 'hypnotherapy' point has already been described in the section on assessment. If this point has been used by the therapist in the treatment session and has proved to be successful, the patient should be asked to use the point at home. They should lie down with the head supported and a pillow placed either side of the head to support the arms. The bilateral points should be stimulated for about 2 minutes, followed by simply holding them for a further 3 minutes, or for as long as it takes to complete the treatment. The patient should be encouraged to visualize what emotion is being highlighted at this moment. It will probably be 'sadness' or 'hopelessness' or something similar. This emotion should be dwelled on for about 5 seconds before 'dropping down' to another emotional layer. The patient simply asks of him or herself 'What lies under this emotion?' or 'What is the cause of this emotion?'. They should be asked to keep the mind fairly blank and to accept the very first thought that enters the head – the emotion may not be the one that is expected. Each 'layer' that is dropped through should last for no more that a few seconds; do *not* linger on each one. It could be detrimental to the treatment and defeat the object of doing it. The emotion of fear is often highlighted after about three or four layers. Fear often lies at the root cause of many emotional disturbances. Once the fear layer has been visualized and passed, the thoughts will often clear to more positive ones. They often change to 'peace', 'joy', 'abundance' etc. When the patient is bathed in positive thoughts and has exhausted the different emotions that he or she is feeling, this is the opportune time to do all manner of things with the thought processes. Visualization is a complicated and varied topic and each person is a unique individual with different needs. It is therefore beyond the scope of this book to suggest how the treatment can be furthered. Suffice it to say, the services of a professional hypnotherapist or psychotherapist are invaluable. What acupressure does is to enhance the procedure by supplying the best acupoint to enable visualization to work better. It would be an excellent idea for the therapist to try this technique on himself or herself before suggesting it for the patient to do. The above technique may be used in the treatment of other emotional disturbances, e.g. anxiety, depression, panic and irritability etc.

4. The energy point in this condition is Ki 6. This point is located just distal to the medial malleolus. It is the very best point for maintaining the energy in the lung channel that has been gained with the treatment. This is an essential component of the session; otherwise the lung energy may start to deplete between one session and another. Ki 6 is also, of course, an excellent point used in stimulating kidney energy, which will help in combating fear and tension.

5. Finally, the body's general energy should be balanced via the Yin component of the Sheng cycle.

Non-acupressure treatment

Sadness and grief often go hand in hand with depression. It is therefore advisable that St John's wort is taken regularly. Homoeopathic Ignatia (made from the St Ignatius Bean) is an excellent remedy to take in both acute and chronic grief. It is best taken in the 30th potency about every hour or so during the day of, say, a funeral and taken once a day to combat chronic melancholy. The taking of Arg. Nit 30 should help anticipation of events that cause distress.

This short chapter has, hopefully, highlighted the efficacy of using acupressure in the treatment of mental and emotional conditions. Emotional imbalance is often the root cause of many physical, organic and hormonal conditions. This huge topic will be further discussed in future publications.

Happy stimulating!

References

Academy of Traditional Chinese Medicine (1975) *An Outline of Chinese Acupuncture*. Foreign Language Press, Beijing.

Boericke, W. (1978) *Homoeopathic Materia Medica*. B. Jain Publishers, New Delhi.

Charman, R.A. (2000) *Complementary Therapies for Physical Therapists*. Butterworth-Heinemann, Oxford.

Cross, J. (1986) *The Relationship of the Chakra Energy System and Acupuncture*. Doctoral Thesis. Copyright held by British College of Acupuncture.

Cross, J. (2000) *Acupressure: Clinical Applications in Musculo-skeletal Conditions*. Butterworth-Heinemann, Oxford.

Cross, J. (in preparation) *Acupressure and Reflextherapy – Healing with the Chakra Energy System*.

Ebner, M. (1962) *Connective Tissue Massage – Theory and Therapeutic Application*. E. and S. Livingstone Ltd, Edinburgh.

Ellis, N. (1994) *Acupuncture in Clinical Practice*. Chapman & Hall, London.

Gach, M.R. (1990) *Acupressure – How to Cure Common Ailments the Natural Way*. Piatkus Publishing, London.

Gallo, F.P and Vincenzi, H. (2000) *Energy Tapping*. New Harbinger Publications, Oakland, California.

Grinberg, A. (1989) *Holistic Reflexology*. Thorsons Publishing Group, Wellingborough, Northants.

Jarmey, C. (1999) *Shiatsu – Foundation Course*. Godsfield Press, Alresford, Hants.

Low, R. (1988) *The Non-meridial Points of Acupuncture*. Thorsons Publishing Group, Wellingborough, Northants.

Maciocia, G. (1989) *The Foundations of Chinese Medicine*. Churchill Livingstone, London.

Shapiro, D. (1996) *Your Body Speaks Your Mind*. Piatkus Publishing, London.

Stormer, C. (1995) *Reflexology – The Definitive Guide*. Hodder and Stoughton, London.

Thie, J.F. (1979) *Touch For Health – A New Approach to Restoring our Natural Energies*. DeVorss and Co., California.

Thompson, W.H. (1985) *Personalysed Diagnosis – Alternative Medicine.* Published privately.

Veith, I. (1972) *The Yellow Emperor's Classic of Internal Medicine.* California Press.

Williams, T. (1996) *Complete Chinese Medicine – A Comprehensive System for Health and Fitness*. Element Books, Bath.

Index